FLETCHERISM
WHAT IT IS

OR

HOW I BECAME YOUNG
AT SIXTY

BY

HORACE FLETCHER A.M.

Fellow American Association for the Advancement of Science

CONTENTS

INTRODUCTION

Fletcherism has become a fact.

A dozen years ago it was laughed at as the "chew-chew" cult; to-day the most famous men of Science endorse it and teach its principles. Scientific leaders at the world's foremost Universities—Cambridge, England; Turin, Italy; Berne, Switzerland; La Sorbonne, France; Berlin, Prussia; Brussels, Belgium; St. Petersburg, Russia; as well as Harvard, Yale and Johns Hopkins in America—have shown themselves in complete accord with Mr. Fletcher's teachings.

The intention of the present volume is that it shall stand as a compact statement of the Gospel of Fletcherism, whereas his other volumes treat the subject more at length and are devoted to different phases of Mr. Fletcher's philosophy. The author here relates briefly the story of his regeneration, of how he rescued himself from the prospect of an early grave, and brought himself to his present splendid physical and mental condition. He tells of the discovery of his principles, which have helped millions of people to live better, happier, and healthier lives.

Mr. Fletcher writes with all his well-known literary charm and vivacity, which have won for his works such a wide-spread popular demand.

It is safe to say that no intelligent reader will peruse this work without becoming convinced that Mr. Fletcher's principles as to eating and living are the sanest that have ever been propounded; that Fletcherism demands no heroic sacrifices of the enjoyments that go to make life worth living, but, to the contrary, that the path to Dietetic Righteousness, which Mr. Fletcher would have us tread, must be the pleasantest of all life's pleasant ways.

THE PUBLISHERS

PREFACE

"What is good for the richest man in the world, must be also good for the poorest, and all in between." Daily Express, *London, May 15th, 1913.*

This quotation was apropos of an announcement in the *Evening Mail*, of New York, telling that the Twentieth Century Crœsus and financial philosopher, John D. Rockefeller, had uttered a Confession of his Faith in the fundamental principles of Dietetic Righteousness and General Efficiency as follows:

"Don't gobble your food. Fletcherize, or chew very slowly while you eat. Talk on pleasant topics. Don't be in a hurry. Take time to masticate and cultivate a cheerful appetite while you eat. So will the demon indigestion be encompassed round about and his slaughter complete."

At the time this compendium of physiological and psychological wisdom concerning the source of health, comfort, and happiness came to my notice I was engaged in furnishing my publishers with a "compact statement of the Gospel of Fletcherism," as they call it, and hence the able assistance of Mr. Rockefeller was welcomed most cordially. Here it was in a nutshell, crystallized, compact, refined, monopolized as to brevity of description, masterly, and practically leaving little more to be said.

The Grand Old Man of Democracy in England, William Ewart Gladstone, had had his say on the same subject some years before, and will be known to the future of physiological fitness more permanently on account of his glorification of Head Digestion of food than for his Liberal Statesmanship.

In like manner, Mr. Rockefeller will deserve more gratitude from posterity for having prescribed the secret of highest mental and physical efficiency in thirty-three words, than for the multiple millions he is dedicating to Science and Sociological Betterment.

It will be interesting, however, to seekers after supermanish health and strength to know how the author took the "straight tip" of Mr. Gladstone, and "worked it for all it was worth" until Mr. Rockefeller referred to the process of common-sense involved as "Fletcherizing."

I assure you it is an interesting story. It has taken nearly fifteen years to bring the development to the point where Mr. Rockefeller, who is carefulness personified when it comes to committing himself for publication, is willing to express his opinion on the subject. It has cost the author unremitting, completely-absorbing, and prayerful concentration of attention, and nearly twenty thousand pounds sterling ($100,000), spent in fostering investigations and securing publicity of the results of the inquiries, with some of the best people in Science, Medicine, and Business helping him with generous assistance, to accomplish this triumph of natural sanity.

In addition to other co-operation, and the most effective, perhaps, it is appropriate to say that there is scarcely a periodical published in all the world, either technical, news-bearing, or otherwise, on the staff of which there has not been some member who has not received some personal benefit from the suggestions carried by the economic system now embodied in the latest dictionaries of many nations as "Fletcherism."

The first rule of "Fletcherism" is to feel gratitude and to express appreciation for and of all the blessings which Nature, intelligence, civilization, and imagination bring to mankind; and this utterance will be endorsed, I am sure, by the millions of persons who have found economy, health, and general happiness through attention to the requirements of dietetic righteousness. It will be especially approved by those who, like Mr. Rockefeller, gained new leases of life after having burned the candle of prudence at both ends and in the middle, to the point of nearly going out, in the struggle for money.

Yet the secret of preserving natural efficiency is even more valuable than cure or repair of damages due to carelessness and over-strain. In this respect the simple rules of Fletcherizing, embodying the requirements of Nature in co-operative nutrition, are made effective by formulating exercises whereby habit-of-conformity is formed, and takes command of the situation so efficiently, that no more thought need be given to the matter than is necessary in regard to breathing, quenching thirst, or observing "the rule of the road" in avoiding collisions in crowded public thoroughfares.

Mr. Rockefeller's thirty-three words not only comprise the practical gist of Fletcherism, but also state the most important fact, that by these means the real dietetic devil, the devil of devils, is kept at a safe distance.

The mechanical act of mastication is easy to manage; but this is not all there is to head digestion. Bad habits of inattention and indifference have to be conquered before good habits of deliberation and appreciation are formed. These requirements of healthy nutrition have been studied extensively and analyzed thoroughly, to the end that we know that they may be acquired with ease if sought with serious interest and respect.

I began the preface by quoting the statement that "What is good for the *richest man in the world* must be also good for the poorest, and all in between." I will close by asserting that

"Doing the right thing in securing right nutrition is easier than not if you only know how."

FLETCHERISM
WHAT IT IS

CHAPTER I

HOW I BECAME A FLETCHERITE

My Turning Point—How I had Ignored My Responsibility—What Happens during Mastication—The Four Principles of Fletcherism

Over twenty years ago, at the age of forty years, my hair was white; I weighed two hundred and seventeen pounds (about fifty pounds more than I should for my height of five feet six inches); every six months or so I had a bad attack of "influenza"; I was harrowed by indigestion; I was afflicted with "that tired feeling." I was an old man at forty, on the way to a rapid decline.

It was at about this time that I applied for a life-insurance policy, and was "turned down" by the examiners as a "poor risk." This was the final straw. I was not afraid to die; I had long ago learned to look upon death with equanimity. At the same time I had a keen desire to live, and then and there made a determination that I would find out what was the matter, and, if I could do so, save myself from my threatened demise.

I realised that the first thing to do was, if possible, to close up my business arrangements so that I could devote myself to the study of how to keep on the face of the earth for a few more years. This I found it possible to do, and I retired from active money-making.

The desire of my life was to live in Japan, where I had resided for several years, and to which country I was passionately devoted. My tastes were in the direction of the fine arts. Japan had been for years my Mecca—my household goods were already there, waiting until I should take up my permanent residence; and it required no small amount of will-power to turn away from the cherished hope of a lifetime, to continue travelling over the world, and concentrate upon finding a way to keep alive.

I turned my back on Japan, and began my quest for health. For a time, I tried some of the most famous "cures" in the world. Here and there were moments of hope, but in the end I was met with disappointment.

THE TURNING POINT

It was partly accidental and partly otherwise that I finally found a clue to the solution of my health disabilities. A faint suggestion of possibilities of arrest of decline had dawned upon me in the city of Galveston, Texas, some years before, and had been strengthened by a visit to an Epicurean philosopher who had a snipe estate among the marshlands of Southern Louisiana and a truffle preserve near Pau, in France. He was a disciple of Gladstone, and faithfully followed the rules relative to thorough chewing of food which the Grand Old Man of England had formulated for the guidance of his children. My friend in Louisiana attributed his robustness of health as much to this protection against overeating as to the exercise incident to his favourite sports. But these impressions had not been strong enough to have a lasting effect.

One day, however, I was called to Chicago to attend to some unfinished business affairs. They were difficult of settlement, and I was compelled to "mark time" in the Western city with nothing especially to do. It was at this time, in 1898, that I began to think seriously of eating and its effect upon health. I read a great many books, only to find that no two authors agreed; and I argued from this fact that no one had found the truth, or else there would be some consensus of agreement. So I stopped reading, and determined to consult Mother Nature herself for direction.

HOW I HAD IGNORED MY RESPONSIBILITY

I began by trying to find out why Nature required us to eat, and how and when. The key to my search was a firm belief in the good intentions of Nature in the interest of our health and happiness, and a belief also that anything less than good health and high efficiency was due to transgressions against certain good and beneficent laws. Hence, it was merely a question of search to find out the nature of the transgression.

The fault was one of nutrition, evidently.

I argued that if Nature had given us personal responsibility it was not hidden away in the dark folds and coils of the alimentary canal where we could not control it. The fault or faults must be committed before the food was swallowed. I felt instinctively that here was the key to the whole situation. The point, then, was to study the cavity of the mouth; and the first thought was: "What happens there?" and "What is present there?" The answer was: Taste, Smell (closely akin to taste and hardly to be distinguished from it), Feeling, Saliva, Mastication, Appetite, Tongue, Teeth, etc.

I first took up the careful study of Taste, necessitating keeping food in the mouth as long as possible, to learn its course and development; and, as I tried it myself, wonders of new and pleasant sensations were revealed. New delights of taste were discovered. Appetite assumed new leanings. Then came the vital discovery, which is this: I found that each of us has what I call a food-filter: a discriminating muscular gate located at the back of the mouth where the throat is shut off from the mouth during the process of mastication. Just where the tongue drops over backward toward its so-called roots there are usually five (sometimes seven, we are told) little teat-like projections placed in the shape of a horseshoe, each of them having a trough around it, and in these troughs, or depressions, terminate a great number of taste-buds, or ends of gustatory nerves. Just at this point the roof of the mouth, or the "hard palate," ends; and the "soft palate," with the uvula at the end of it, drops down behind the heavy part of the tongue.

During the natural act of chewing the lips are closed, and there is also a complete closure at the back part of the mouth by the pressing of the tongue against the roof of the mouth. During mastication, then, the mouth is an airtight pouch.

After which brief description, please note, the next time you take food,

WHAT HAPPENS DURING MASTICATION

Hold the face down, so that the tongue hangs perpendicularly in the mouth. This is for two reasons: one, because it will show how food, when properly mixed with saliva, will be lifted up in the hollow part in the middle of the tongue, against the direct force of gravity, and will collect at the place where the mouth is shut off at the back, the food-gate.

It is a real gate; and while the food is being masticated, so that it may be mixed with saliva and chemically transformed from its crude condition into the chemical form that makes it possible of digestion and absorption, this gate will remain tightly shut, and the throat will be entirely cut off from the mouth.

But as the food becomes creamy, so to speak, through being mixed with saliva, or emulsified, or alkalised, or neutralised, or dextrinised, or modified in whatever form Nature requires, the creamy substance will be drawn up the central conduit of the tongue until it reaches the food-gate.

If it is found by the taste-buds there located around the "circumvalate papillæ" (the teat-like projections on the tongue which I mentioned above) to be properly prepared for acceptance and further digestion, the food-gate will open, and the food thus ready for acceptance into the body will be sucked back and swallowed unconsciously—that is, without conscious effort.

I now started to experiment on myself. I chewed my food carefully until I extracted all taste from it there was in it, and until it slipped unconsciously down my throat. When the appetite ceased, and I was thereby told that I had had enough, I stopped; and I had no desire to eat any more until a real appetite commanded me again. Then I again chewed carefully—eating always whatever the appetite craved.

THE FIVE PRINCIPLES OF FLETCHERISM

I have now found out five things; all that there is to my discovery relative to optimum nutrition; and to the fundamental requisite of what is called Fletcherism.

First: Wait for a true, earned appetite.

Second: Select from the food available that which appeals most to appetite, and in the order called for by appetite.

Third: Get all the good taste there is in food out of it in the mouth, and swallow only when it practically "swallows itself."

Fourth: Enjoy the good taste for all it is worth, and do not allow any depressing or diverting thought to intrude upon the ceremony.

Fifth: Wait; take and *enjoy as much as possible* what appetite approves; Nature will do the rest.

For five months I went on patiently observing, and I found out positively in that time that I had worked out my own salvation. I had lost upwards of sixty pounds of fat: I was feeling better in all ways than I had for twenty years. My head was clear, my body felt springy, I enjoyed walking, I had not had a single cold for five months, "that tired feeling" was gone! But my skin had not yet shrunk back to fit my reduced proportions, and when I told friends whom I met that I felt well and a new man, their retort was that I certainly "did not look it!"[A]

The more I tried to convince others, the more fully I realised from talking to friends how futile and well-nigh hopeless was the attempt to get credence and sympathy for my beliefs, scientifically well founded as I felt they were. For years it proved so; and I faced the fact that to pursue the campaign for recognition meant spending much money, putting aside opportunities to make profit in other and more agreeable directions, and no end of ridicule. Sometimes, during the daytime, when I was "sizing up" the situation in my mind, treating it with calm business judgment, it seemed nothing less than insane to waste any more time or money in trying to prove my contentions.

Fully three years passed before I received encouragement from any source of recognised authority. I went first to Professor Atwater,[B] who received me most politely, but when I told him my story he threw cold water on my enthusiasm. In our correspondence afterwards he was most cordial but in no way encouraging.

The frost became more and more repellent and benumbing.

Still I persisted. At last I got hold of my first convert: a medical man, ill and discouraged; a member of a family long distinguished in the medical profession. He was Doctor Van Someren, of Venice, Italy, where I had made my home and where I lived for some years. I induced him to organise an experiment with me. We enlisted a squad of men and induced them to take food according to my ideas. We also were fortunate enough to secure the co-operation of Professor Leonardi, of Venice.

In less than three weeks the sick physician found himself relieved of his acute ailments, and it would have taken several teams of horses to hold him back from preaching his discovery.[C] A little later, we transferred the field of experiment to the Austrian Tyrol, and tested our endurance qualities, only to find a capacity for work that was not before considered possible. Then Doctor Van Someren wrote his paper for the British Medical Association, which excited the interest of Professor Sir Michael Foster, of the University of Cambridge, England, and the first wave of scientific attention was set in motion.

CHAPTER II

SCIENTIFIC TESTS

First Critical Examination at Cambridge University, England—My Endurance Test at Yale University in America

One result of this powerful interest was a test of our theories made at Cambridge University, England, organised by Sir Michael Foster, who was then Professor of Physiology at the University, and conducted by Professor Francis Gowland Hopkins. The test was successful, proving our most optimistic claims, and the report of it was published.

The scientific world now began to turn its attention to my discoveries. Doctor Henry Pickering Bowditch, of Harvard Medical School, the dean of American physiologists, put the full weight of his respected influence into the work to secure for America the honour of completing the investigation; but it was not until the experiments at Yale University, in New Haven, that the first wide publicity was accorded. The story of this and subsequent experiments and their results is this: Professor Russell H. Chittenden was at the time President of the American Physiological Association, Director of the Sheffield Scientific School of Yale

University, and the recognised leading physiological chemist of America. He invited me to the annual meeting of the Physiological Association at Washington, where I described the results in economy and efficiency, and especially in getting rid of fatigue of brain and muscle, obtained up to that time. But evidently to little purpose, as Professor Chittenden revealed to me at the close of the meeting. He said, in effect:

"Fletcher, all the men you have met at our meeting like you immensely, personally; but no one takes much stock in your claims, even with the endorsement of the Cambridge men; the test there was insufficient to be conclusive. If, however, you will come to New Haven and let us put you through an examination, our report will be accepted here. You will be either justified or disillusioned; and—I want to be frank with you—I think you will be disillusioned."

MY EXAMINATION

by Dr. Chittenden showed a daily average of 44.9 grams of proteid, 38.0 grams of fat, and 253 grams of carbohydrates, with a total average calorie value of 1,606 (*compare this with the Voit Diet Standard, page 109*), and careful and thorough tests made at the Yale Gymnasium proved that, in spite of this relatively low ration, I was in prime physical condition.

Previously, as before stated, in the autumn of 1901, Dr. Van Someren had accompanied me to Cambridge for the purpose of having our claims closely investigated, with the assistance of physiological experts. The Cambridge and the Venice findings were fully confirmed at New Haven, and striking physical evidence was added by Doctor William Gilbert Anderson's examinations of me in the Yale Gymnasium. This latter test, described on page 24, was more practically important as an eye-opener to both doctors and laymen than were the laboratory reports. I personally showed endurance and strength in special tests superior to the foremost among the College athletes. This was without training and with comparatively small muscle; the superiority of the muscle lying in the quality and not in the amount of it.

Professor Chittenden then became intensely interested in the matter, as did also Professor Mendel; and the former suggested organising an experiment on a sufficiently large scale to prove universality of application or the reverse. He volunteered his services and the use of his laboratory facilities.

At this time, too, I became acquainted with General Leonard Wood[D] and Surgeon-General O'Reilly, of the United States Army. I found both open to my evidence; and, in the case of General Wood, I learned that it was confirmed by his own experience while chasing Indians in the Western wilds. Through them President Roosevelt and Secretary Root became interested, and *carte blanche* was given General O'Reilly to use the War Department facilities, including the soldiers of the Hospital Corps, for assistance in the proposed experiment.[E]

One of the revelations of our experiments worthy of mention here was that occasional long abstinence from food, say two or three weeks, with water freely available, is comparatively harmless, if "Fletcherizing" is carefully practised when food is again given to the body. Nature prescribes accurately what is to be eaten (often the most unexpected sort of food); and if the food selected by appetite is carefully masticated, sipped, or whatever other treatment is necessary to get the good taste out of it, and the mental state at the same time is clear of fear-thought or worry of any kind, the just amount that the body can use at the moment is prescribed by appetite, and the restoration to normal weight is accomplished with epicurean delight, well worth a spell of deprivation.

THE IRVING FISHER EXPERIMENTS

The tests of endurance, which were conducted by Professor Irving Fisher, of Yale, now President of the Committee of One Hundred on National Health of the American Association for the Advancement of Science, and with the co-operation of the famous athletic coach, Alonzo B. Stagg, formerly of Yale, but now of the University of Chicago—on College athletes, students of sedentary habits, and on members of the staff of the Battle Creek Sanatorium—are of prodigious importance in their relation to the possibilities of human endurance through simple Fletcherizing.

The reports include a test in what is termed "deep-knee bending," or squatting on the heels and then lifting the body to full height as many times as possible. John H. Granger, of the Battle Creek Sanatorium staff, did this feat 5,002 times consecutively in two hours and nineteen minutes and could have continued. He then ran down a flight of steps to the swimming-pool, plunged in and had a swim, slept sweetly and soundly for the usual time, and showed no signs of soreness or other disability afterwards.

Doctor Wagner gave his strenuous contribution to our knowledge of possibilities of endurance by holding his arms out horizontally for 200 minutes without rest— three hours and twenty minutes. At the end of that time he showed no signs of fatigue, and stopped only because of the weariness shown by those who were watching and counting the minutes. These statements seem like exaggerations, but they are not.

Both of these tests can be tried by any one in the privacy of his or her own bedroom.

Doctor Anderson, Director of the Yale Gymnasium, taking advantage of the cue offered by the Yale experiments, which he superintended, practised Fletcherizing in all its branches. At the end of six years he put the muscles thus purified to the test, with the result that he added fifteen pounds of pure muscle to a frame that never carried more than 135 pounds before in the half century of its existence, and demonstrated that the same progressive recuperation that I have enjoyed is open and available to others who have passed middle life.

Mr. Stapleton, one of Professor Chittenden's volunteers, grasped the same valuable cue while serving as one of the heavy-weight test-subjects in the Yale experiments. He reduced his waist measurement to thirty inches and a half, increased his chest measurement to forty-four inches; and has refined his physique until his ribs show clearly through his flesh, while his muscles mount tall and strong where muscle is needed in the economy of efficiency. In the meantime, without training other than that connected with his teaching, he increased the total of his strength and endurance more than one hundred per cent.; and reduced his amount of food by nearly, if not quite, half—as have also Doctor Anderson and myself.

MY ENDURANCE TEST AT YALE

These are merely typical cases of distinguished and measured improvement.

How the movement went on from step to step others have told, and I need not follow it further here.

Two years after I began my experiments my strength and endurance had increased beyond my wildest expectation. On my fiftieth birthday I rode nearly two hundred miles on my bicycle over French roads, and came home feeling fine. Was I stiff the next day? Not at all, and I rode fifty miles the next morning before breakfast in order to test the effect of my severe stunt.[F]

When I was fifty-eight years of age, at the Yale University Gymnasium, under the observation of Dr. Anderson, I lifted three hundred pounds dead weight three hundred and fifty times with the muscles of my right leg below the knee. The record of the best athlete then was one hundred and seventy-five lifts, so I doubled the world's record of that style of tests of endurance.

The story of this test at Yale, when I doubled the "record" about which so much has been written, is this: Professor Irving Fisher, of Yale, had devised a new form of endurance-testing machine intended to be used upon the muscles most commonly in use by all persons. Obviously these are the muscles used in walking. Quite a large number of tests had been measured by the Fisher machine, but it was still being studied with a view to possible simplification.

I was asked to try it and to suggest any changes that might improve it. I did so, and handled the weight with such seeming ease that Dr. Anderson asked me whether I would not make a thorough test of my endurance. This I was glad to do.

The Professor Irving Fisher Endurance Testing Machine is weighted to 75 per cent. of the lifting capacity of the subject, ascertained by means of the Kellog Mercurial Dynamometer. The lifting is timed to the beats of a metronome.

When I began, Dr. Anderson cautioned me against attempting too much. I asked him what he considered "too much," and he replied: "For a man of your age, not in training, I should not recommend trying more than fifty lifts." So I began the test, lifting the weight to the beat of the metronome at the rate of about one in two seconds, and had soon reached the fifty mark. "Be careful," repeated Dr. Anderson, "you may not feel that you are overdoing now, but afterwards you may regret it."

But I felt no strain and went on.

When seventy-five had been exceeded, Dr. Anderson called Dr. Born from his desk to take charge of the counting and watching to see that the lifts were fully completed, and ran out into the gymnasium to call the masters of boxing, wrestling, fencing, etc., to witness the test. When they had gathered about the machine, Dr. Anderson said to them, "It looks as if we were going to see a record-breaking." I then asked, "What are the records?" Dr. Anderson replied, "One hundred and seventy-five lifts is the record; only two men have exceeded one hundred; the lowest was thirty-three, and the average so far is eighty-four."

In the meantime I had reached one hundred and fifty lifts, and the interest was centered on the question as to whether I should reach the high record, one hundred and seventy-five.

When one hundred and seventy-five had been reached, Dr. Anderson stepped forward to catch me in case the leg in use in the test should not be able to support me when I stopped and attempted to stand up. But I did not stop lifting the three-hundred-pound weight. I kept right on, and as I progressed to two hundred, two hundred and fifty, three hundred, and finally to double the record, three hundred and fifty lifts, the interest increased progressively.

After adding a few to the three hundred and fifty I stopped, not because I was suffering from fatigue, but because the pounding of the iron collar on the muscles above my knee had made the place so pummelled very sore, as if hit a great number of times with a heavy sledge-hammer. I had doubled the record, and that seemed sufficient for a starter in the competition.

As I stood up, Dr. Anderson reached up his arms to support me. But I needed no support. The leg that had been in use felt a trifle lighter, but in no sense weak or tired.

Then I was examined for heart-action, steadiness of nerve, muscle, etc., and was found to be all right, with no evidence of strain. A glass brimming full of water was placed first in one hand and then in the other, and was held out at arm's length without spilling any of the water.

Next morning I was examined for evidence of soreness, but none was present. There was the normal elasticity and tone of muscle.

Later in that same year, at the International Young Men's Christian Association Training School at Springfield, Massachusetts, I lifted seven hundred and seventy pounds with the muscles of the back and legs—a feat that weight-lifting athletes find hard to perform. And I did these stunts eating two meals a day, one at noon and the other at six o'clock, at an average cost of eleven cents a day.

Still another examination at the University of Pennsylvania resulted in my breaking the College record of lifting power with the back muscles. I do not cite these instances as feats of extraordinary prowess, but just to show the difference in my condition then and twenty years before. All this I have done simply by keeping my body free of excess of food and the poisons that come from the putrefaction of the food that the organism does not want and cannot take care of.

As to myself, I am now past sixty-four. I weigh one hundred and seventy pounds, which is a good weight for my height. During the many years of experiment I have ranged between two hundred and seventeen and one hundred and thirty pounds, but have "settled down" to my present quite convenient figure. I feel perfectly well; I can do as much work as can a man of forty—more than can the average man of forty, I believe. I rarely have a cold, and although I am always careless in this regard, my work is never delayed. I do not know what it is to have "that tired feeling," except as expressed by sleepiness. When I get into bed I scarce ever remember my head striking the pillow, and after four and one-half hours I awake from a dreamless slumber with a happy waking thought in process of formation.

I usually find it agreeable to court supplemental naps, to be followed by more pleasant waking thoughts: but these are pure luxury. I can do with five hours sleep if need be.

CHAPTER III

WHAT I AM ASKED ABOUT FLETCHERISM

Let Nature Choose the Meals—How Many Meals a Day?—Housewives—Fletcherism—The Financial Economy of Fletcherism—Business People and Fletcherism—The True Epicure

What do I eat?

When do I eat?

How much do I eat?

My answer to all these questions is very simple. I eat anything that my appetite calls for; I eat it only when it *does* call for it; and I eat until my appetite is satisfied and cries "Enough!"

With my New England food preferences, my range of selection circulates among a very simple and inexpensive variety, namely, potatoes, corn-bread, beans, occasionally eggs, milk, cream, toast-and-butter, etc.; and combinations of these, such as hashed-browned potatoes, potatoes in cream, potatoes *au gratin*, baked potatoes, potato pats, fish-balls—mainly composed of potato; occasionally tomato stewed with plenty of powdered sugar; oyster stew with the flavour of celery; escalloped oysters, etc. The taste for fruits is always suitable to the season, and is intermittent, strong leanings towards some particular fruit persisting for a time and then waning to give place to some other preference.

But with all my fifteen or twenty years of unremitting study of the subject, I cannot now tell what my body is going to want to-morrow. But Nature knows, and she alone knows.

LET NATURE CHOOSE THE MEAL

Once in Venice a group of experimenters, of which I was one, subsisted on milk alone. During seventeen days nothing but milk, always from the same cow, and fresh from the milking, passed my lips in the way of food or drink. I sipped the milk, and tasted it for all the taste there was in it, and I learned to be so fond of it that it was with some difficulty that I went back to a varied diet when the experiment called for a change. Good, fresh milk is an exception to Nature's dislike for monotony in food. Milk is the one perfectly-balanced food material; and while it may not be always the best food for grown persons, it is the most acceptable as a monotonous diet, and always is good, sufficient and safe nutriment, if sipped, tasted, and naturally swallowed.

I have forgotten just what the exact quantity was that I consumed daily during those seventeen days—I believe it was about two quarts. I get away as far as possible from quantitative amounts, which may influence other persons. The appetite is the only true guide to bodily need; and if milk is tasted and swallowed only by involuntary compulsion as required by right feeding, the appetite will gauge the bodily need exactly, and cut off short when enough for the moment has been taken.

So I say to all who ask me these questions as applied to themselves: I cannot advise you appropriately what to eat, when to eat, nor how much to eat; neither can anybody else. Trust to Nature absolutely, and accept her guidance.

If she calls for pie, eat pie. If she calls for it at midnight eat it then, but eat it right. Understand the food filter at the back of the mouth as I have described it in a previous article, and use it in connection with the pie. If it is used properly, and all the taste is extracted from the pie, and it is swallowed only in response to the natural opening of the gate, and if the ingredients of the pie that are not swallowed naturally are removed from the mouth, nothing will happen to disturb profound sleep.

Few persons will crave mince pie or Welsh rarebit late at night. The worker on a morning paper may do so, and often does. He has earned his appetite, and sometimes it is so robust as to call for mince pie or Welsh rarebit; but if these are eaten properly they will then be utilised by the body, eagerly and easily.

I dwell purposely upon this extravagance of eating. It is to accentuate the fact that we want to get as far away as possible, when cultivating vital economies, from the idea of extraneous advice in the matter of food.

The ordinary person will probably find his appetite leaning towards the simplest of foods, and away from frequency of indulgence. If the breakfast is postponed until a real, earned appetite has been secured, the mid-day or later breakfast (remember always that breakfast means the first meal of the day, no matter when taken) will be so enjoyable a meal, and the appetite will be so entirely satisfied that there will be no more demand for food until evening, and possibly not even then.

HOW MANY MEALS A DAY?

I am often asked if it is true that I eat only two meals a day; that I never eat breakfast, and why I have dropped that meal.

I have two meals a day more habitually than any other number, but not with any prescribed regularity, for the reason that my activities are most irregular at times, and my appetite accommodates itself to my needs.

When I am doing work under the most favourable of conditions, one meal a day is the rhythm best appreciated by my body. But the question of "How many meals a day?" is tantamount to the inquiry as to the amount of sleep needed: it is a matter of satisfaction of the natural requirements. The harder one works, the faster one runs, etc., the more air he needs. The same applies to the need for food according to the amount of heat eliminated, and the repair material consumed. The really hardest work that anybody does is done within the body. Muscular effort in normal conditions is not so waste-provoking and exacting as getting rid of excess of food and the counteraction of worry or anger. Likewise, idleness begets uneasiness, uneasiness begets desire for something (nobody knows just what), and groping around for "Don't know what" causes the temptation to eat and drink something which the body does not need; and then the really hard work of the body begins in the attempt of Nature to get rid of the excess. Excess of water can be thrown off in perspiration with comparative ease, but with excess of food it is different. The kidneys, bacteria and fuel furnaces of the body are all over-worked to get rid of it.

When I am so busy that I have only time to replenish the real exhausted need of the body, say half an hour at most, I find one meal a day all that my appetite demands of me. This is taken after I have done my day's work of, say, eight hours of writing, or twelve or thirteen hours of bicycle riding or mountain climbing, and then I do not have appetite for more until the next day, after the work is done.

When I mention two meals as being the more habitual, it is because I am not fully, constructively active all the time now, although I am usually "snowed under" with things that I *might* do to advantage; and hence I conform to the social custom and sit down to table some time in the evening to be social.

The reason I have dropped the habit-hunger morning meal is because I find that it is unnatural in my case. My experience showed me that omission of the early morning meal led to desire for a lighter but more satisfactory mid-day meal, and took away the craving for the evening supper. I first came to this realisation during excessive hot weather and monotonously trying environment. The only time I could write comfortably was before sun-up in the morning. Absorbed in my writing I did not realise the growing heat of the day until I actually began to rain perspiration, by which time it was nearly noon. Then came the mid-day meal of breakfast selection with salad and fruit preponderating. The best of feelings followed, the waist-line shrank, and one meal satisfied.

In order to try the urgency of any habit appetite—the early morning meal, for instance—take a drink of water instead, and note if that does not suffice as well as food to allay the craving for "something." A cup of hot water, with sugar and milk to suit the taste, is amply sufficient. Water will not satisfy a real, earned appetite; but it often will effectually allay a purely habit-hunger such as that for early breakfast.

HOUSEWIVES AND FLETCHERISM

A great many women ask: "But how is it possible to follow such a haphazard way of eating in a home without upsetting the whole routine of the household, disturbing the work of the servants? You can't just have your family eating whenever they like."

My answer is this: The possible disturbance to domestic regularity and convenience, because of the difficulty of supplying different members of the family only when appetite in each case is "just good and ready," is purely imaginary. Persons of regular occupations will accommodate themselves to the ordinary rhythm of meal schedule easily and naturally, with the difference that they may occasionally skip a meal or two when the ordinary activity has been lessened.

The general experience has been, that concentration on one particular meal, either at noon or in the evening, will suit everybody, and other feedings will be "snoopings" from the larder, or taken at a restaurant in those instances where one's occupation is remote from home. The "Fletcherite" at business frequently follows the method of having nuts or plain biscuits in his desk in case he feels like taking them; and the business woman would do well to profit by his example.

The adoption of Fletcheristic simplicity leads to the solving of the eternal household problem, and under its influence it is possible for woman's work to be done sooner, giving physical relief and more time for healthful recreation.

Diminution of the demand for meat-foods has much to do with both the ease of house-work, and the modification of cost. But this is not the most important saving. The saving of liability to intestinal toxication (poisoning) is the great economy of the method.

THE FINANCIAL ECONOMY OF FLETCHERISM

It has been stated by writers who have correctly reported results that more than two hundred thousand families in America live according to Fletcherism and save as much as a dollar a day on their living expenses. This has led many to ask: "How are one's living expenses reduced by your principles?"

The estimate, arrived at a few years ago, that some two hundred thousand families in America were saving an average of a dollar a day through Fletcherizing, was made, I believe, by Doctor Kellog, of Battle Creek, Michigan. Through the thousands of patients who pass under his observation, and through a comprehensive touch with the sale of different kinds of food throughout the country, Doctor Kellog has his finger on the pulse of the nation in relation to its dietetic circulation. Fletcherism first affected families of sumptuous tastes, and the economy of it easily effected a saving of an average of a dollar a day, largely in the diminution of meat requirements and complex dishes.

The spread of the movement has now begun to encompass families of lesser luxury of habits; and here it is found that an average saving of ten cents a day for each person is easily accomplished. In the Christian Endeavour Society alone, the leaders of the movement, as the result of their own practical experience, hoped to effect a saving of hundreds of thousands of dollars a day through the spread of this economic nutritive teaching. This was likewise the aspiration of the Roman Catholic benevolent organisations. A circular letter signed by the Reverend Father Higgins, of Germantown, Pennsylvania, which was distributed widely, declared that, in addition to the food economy sought to be obtained, a condition which makes for poverty—that is, intemperance—was overcome by Fletcherism.

Father Higgins declared that "*No Fletcherite can be intemperate in the use of alcoholic stimulants,*" and he was right in his assertion.

BUSINESS PEOPLE AND FLETCHERISM

What would be the best way for business people to adopt Fletcherism? is often asked. The case is frequently cited to me of a young man or woman who isn't hungry for breakfast at seven o'clock, does not eat at that time because the appetite doesn't demand it; and then gets ravenously hungry at eleven o'clock. It may be impossible to get any food until one-thirty—by which time the feeling comes that one has "waited too long," and a headache and no desire for food are the results. Or, the case of working-girls who live in boarding-houses, eat no breakfast, and at noon cannot afford the wholesome and hearty food Nature would then crave. Later, at dinner, they have to eat what is put before them, whether they want it or not, or else go without. Will a hearty luncheon, rightly eaten, interfere with a good afternoon's work? I am reminded also that leisure, money, and easily-accessible cafés are not always available for business women.

My answer to such questions is:—Any change of habit is apt to excite a protest on behalf of the body, especially when the body is not properly nourished, and is in a state of more or less disease. When the habit-hunger comes on a few sips of water will quiet the discomfort for the time being and, very likely, until it is convenient to take food comfortably and with the calm and relish necessary to good digestion. Headache, faintness, "all-goneness" and like discomforts, are symptoms, not of hunger, but of the reverse—that is, fermentation of undigested excess of food which the body cannot use.

A person, thus troubled, should brave discomfort for a week, and even go without food entirely for a few meals, in order to give the body a chance to "clean house": then the real sensation of hunger will be expressed by "watering of the mouth" and a keen desire for some simple food such as bread and butter, or dry bread alone. But this healthy appetite will "keep" and accumulate until it is convenient to take food.

THE TRUE EPICURE

I am, personally, a hearty man in full activity, both mental and physical. I can work six hours and then satisfy the keenest of appetites on a meal of wheat griddle-cakes with maple syrup and a glass or two of milk. A young working woman should be able to do the same. If I eat such a meal with "gusto," deliberation (so as to enjoy the maximum of taste), taking not more than fifteen minutes over it, I can then go to work, or play, or to mountain climbing, or to riding a bicycle, and keep it up until I am sleepy, with no sense of repletion or discomfort.

"Money, leisure and easily-accessible cafés" are the menace of right nutrition, unless one is proof against temptation to kill time in this dangerous manner.

Steady work to earn a true appetite, small means to spend on food, the necessity of going to seek it, with the appreciation which comes from rarity, are the very best safeguards to right nutrition.

I am an epicure. Yet I have never seen a boarding-house, nor a restaurant, nor a camp where I could not find something to satisfy a true (earned) appetite. During more than a year in the Far East—Ceylon, Java, the Philippines, China, Burma, India, Kashmir—and at many steamer and railway lunch tables, I always found something good to satisfy a keen appetite. If you are all right inside, and will only conquer your habit-hungers, I believe you can live sumptuously, anywhere, on less than two shillings a day. I can, and often do; and do it, too, at one hundred and seventy pounds weight and "awfully busy" all the time. It may be difficult, and perhaps painful, at first, to get the best of bad habit-cravings, but it is worth while. A week should accomplish the reformation.

A number of men ask me: "Do you honestly believe that in your theories lies the secret of long life?" I do, and I may give one example of a "lived model" of longevity as the result of Fletcherism in all its ramifications of temperance of eating, careful mastication, radiant optimism, practical altruism, superabundant activity, etc. The Honourable Albert Gallatin Dow, of Randolph, New York, passed away in May, 1908, lacking less than three months of a hundred years of age. Up to the last moment of his century of life there was no encroachment of senility, and he fell, ripe fruit, into the lap of Mother Nature, without a blemish of decay. Shortly before he passed away, Mr. Dow invited me to see him, and told me that he had received a shock of warning early in life as I had done late in life, and had made the same discovery that had reformed me. He believed that he owed his health and vigour to following the simple requirements of Nature, as I was teaching; but he had his career to make at the time, and had not had the leisure and means to preach dietetic righteousness as I was doing. He wished me Godspeed on my mission. All inquiry in all directions, wherever longevity has been accomplished, reveals the same simplicity of habits of living, which are the natural points of Fletcherizing.

CHAPTER IV

RULES OF FLETCHERISM

Never Eat until Hungry—Mouth-Treatment of Solid and Liquid Food—When to Stop Eating—Instructions to the Medical Department of the U. S. Army

To make my ideas a little clearer, I will elaborate them a little more. Remember that the rules are exceedingly simple. That, to my mind, is the worst obstruction to the general adoption of my system: it is so simple that many find it difficult to comprehend. But take these rules and you have the idea.

FIRST RULE

Don't take any food until you are "good and hungry."

Some people will reply: "I am always hungry." Others will aver that they "never know what it is to be hungry." We may assume that both replies are incorrect, because hunger must be intermittent, and must sometimes be present, or life would be intolerable through lack of satisfaction and something to satisfy.

The question, "What is hunger?" is a natural and legitimate one, for the reason that there are true appetites and false cravings. True hunger for food is indicated by "watering of the mouth"—not that watering of the mouth, or profuse flow of saliva, through artificial excitement by some pungent stimulant, such as sweets, or acids or spiced things; but that which is excited on thought of some of the simplest of foods, such as bread and butter, or dry bread alone.

"All-goneness" in the region of the stomach, "faintness," or any of the discomforts that are felt below the guillotine line, are not signs of true hunger, but symptoms of indigestion, or some other form of disease. True hunger is never a discomfort unless a growing desire may be classed as a discomfort. Accumulating appetite (true hunger) is like the multiplication of uncut and uncashed coupons on a railway bond or on a Government bond. The feeling of possession is a joy of itself; and the ability to collect the proceeds when needed and at leisure is comfortable rather than uncomfortable. Under circumstances of intelligent nutrition, if we pass one meal-time we wait patiently for the next, with the knowledge that we are accumulating appetite coupons.

SECOND RULE

Have you yet learned what true hunger is?

Don't go on unless you have done so. Take a little more time; skip a meal or two, and give Nature a chance to show you what real appetite (true watering of the mouth) is. Having learned to recognise healthy hunger and appetite, and to know what it is to have both of them begging you for satisfaction, proceed with the second rule.

From the food available at the time take that first which appeals most strongly to the appetite. It may be a sip of soup, or a bite of bread and butter, or a nibble of cheese, or, perhaps a lump of sugar. It may be a piece of meat, though I doubt that a true appetite will call for such at the beginning of a meal. Never mind what it may be, give it a trial. If it be something that should be masticated in order to give the saliva a chance to mix with it and chemically transform it, chew it "for all that it is worth."

"For all that it is worth" means for the extraction and enjoyment of all the good taste there is in it.

If the food selected by the appetite happens to be soup, or milk, or some mushy substance, get all the good taste out of it, doing all you can to accomplish this; for to get the taste out of food is an assurance of digesting it, and the pleasure it gives in the process of Nature's way of getting you to do the right thing in helping her to nourish yourself properly. Sip, taste, bite, press with the tongue against the roof of the mouth, the food in the mouth, not because of any suggestion of mine, but in response to the natural instinct to move it about and get out of it all the taste there is in it.

THIRD RULE

The moment appetite begins to slack up a bit, the moment saliva does not flow so freely as at first, the moment there is any degree of satisfaction of the appetite, stop eating!

You will have a return of appetite; you will have another chance to eat; appetite is beginning to have "that tired feeling" herself; be kind to her as she has been kind to you. Give her a rest! Give her a rest! Give yourself a rest! Rest is the antidote of "that tired feeling"! Therefore rest the appetite before it gets tired. Stop eating before you are overloaded.

Now, having learned how to do the right thing in eating so as never more to have "that tired feeling," don't begin to overdo. Don't bend backward too far. Don't ever overdo a good thing.

Be temperate; be deliberate. Be thoughtful; be forethoughtful; be forethoughtful without being fearthoughtful. Don't overdo chewing, for then you take away much of the pleasure; smother the psychic enjoyment of eating, and raise the very mischief again.

Just be natural, and know that being natural is being deliberate in enjoying the thing you are doing, for that is Nature's way.

To the above simple rules I will append a few recommendations which occurred to me and which I wrote while in a respiration calorimeter, an experience which I will relate in a subsequent chapter. This list of recommendations has since been included in the Instructions to the Medical Department of the United States Army, under the heading:

Method of attaining Economic Assimilation of Nutriment and Immunity from Disease, Muscular Soreness and Fatigue.

(1) Feed only when a distinct appetite has been earned.

(2) Masticate all solid food until it is completely liquefied and excites in an irresistible manner the swallowing reflex or swallowing impulse.

(3) Attention to the act and appreciation of the taste are necessary, meantime, to excite the flow of gastric juice into the stomach to meet the food—as demonstrated by Pawlow.

(4) Strict attention to these two particulars will fulfil the requirements of Nature relative to the preparation of the food for digestion and assimilation; and this being faithfully done, the automatic processes of digestion and assimilation will proceed most profitably, and will result in discarding very little digestion-ash (fæces) to encumber the intestines, or to compel excessive draft upon the body energy for excretion.

(5) The assurance of healthy economy is observed in the small amount of excreta and its peculiar inoffensive character, showing escape from putrid bacterial decomposition such as brings indol and skatol offensively into evidence.

(6) When digestion and assimilation has been normally economic, the digestion-ash (fæces) may be formed into little balls ranging in size from a pea to a so-called Queen Olive, according to the food taken, and should be quite dry, having only the odour of moist clay or of a hot biscuit. This inoffensive character remains indefinitely until the ash completely dries, or disintegrates like rotten stone or wood.

(7) The weight of the digestive-ash may range (moist) from 10 grams to not more than 40-50 grams a day, according to the food; the latter estimate being based on a vegetarian diet, and may not call for excretion for several days; smallness indicating best condition. Foods differ so materially that the amount and character of the excreta cannot be accurately specified. Some foods and conditions demand two evacuations daily. Thorough and faithful Fletcherizing settles the question satisfactorily.

(8) Fruits may hasten peristalsis[G]; but not if they are treated in the mouth as sapid liquids rather than as solids, and are insalivated, sipped, tasted, into absorption in the same way wine-tasters test and take wine, and tea-tasters test tea. The latter spit out the tea after tasting, as, otherwise, it vitiates their taste, and ruins them for their discriminating profession.

(9) Milk, soups, wines, beer, and all sapid liquids or semi-solids should be treated in this manner for the best assimilation and digestion as well as for the best gustatory results.

(10) This would seem to entail a great deal of care and bother, and lead to a waste of time.

(11) Such, however, is not the case. To give attention in the beginning does require strict attention and persistent care to overcome life-long habits of nervous haste; but if the attack is earnest, habits of careful mouth treatment and appetite discrimination soon become fixed, and cause deliberation in taking food unconsciously to the feeder.

(12) Food of a proteid value of 5-7 grams of nitrogen and 1,500-2,500 calories of fuel value,[H] paying strict attention to the appetite for selection and carefully treated in the mouth, has been found to be the quantity best suited to economy and efficiency of both mind and body in sedentary pursuits and ordinary business activity; and, also, such habit of economy has given practical immunity from the common diseases for a period extending over more than fifteen years, whereas the same subject was formerly subject to periodical illness. Similar economy and immunity have shown themselves consistently in the cases of many test subjects covering periods of ten years, and applies equally to both sexes, all ages, and other idiosyncratic conditions.

(13) The time necessary for satisfying complete body needs and appetite daily, when the habit of attention, appreciation and deliberation have been installed, is less than half an hour, no matter how divided as to number of rations. This necessitates industry of mastication, to be sure, and will not admit of waste of much time between mouthfuls.

(14) Ten or fifteen minutes will completely satisfy a ravenous appetite if all conditions of ingestion and preparation are favourable.

(15) Both quantitive and qualitive supply of saliva are important factors; but attention to these fundamental requirements of right eating soon regulates the supply of all of the digestive juices, and in connection with the care recommended above, ensures economy of nutrition and, probably, immunity from disease.

CHAPTER V

WHAT IS PROPER MASTICATION?

Not Excessive Chewing—Gladstone's Advice—Salival Action on Starch Foods

Notwithstanding the fact that Fletcherizing stands for tasting as the important thing to accomplish before food is swallowed, and that biting, chewing, or masticating is merely a means to secure the end of thorough tasting, nine-tenths of all who know anything about the claims for Fletcherizing insist on thinking that it merely means "excessive mastication." The National Food Reform Association of England, in a bulletin giving advice concerning the feeding of school children, intended to be posted in school-rooms and private dining rooms, speak of Fletcherizing in its ideal practice as "Excessive Mastication."

This is just what Fletcherizing is not. The very essence of the method of performing the personal responsibility is avoiding excess of anything, excessive or laboured chewing among the rest.

There is little if any harm in keeping food in the mouth as long as possible, and I believe that it is impossible to have too much saliva mixed with it when it is swallowed, because when it is properly tasted and insalivated it is almost impossible to hold it back from the food gate at the back of the mouth. There is always suction there ready to draw welcome nourishment in when it is ready, and readiness touches a button, electrically relieving the muscular springs that close the gate tightly during tasting, and, literally a "team of horses could not hold it."

What the mystics of the stomach-diseases profession called *bradefagy*, or, in plain English, excessive chewing, can only be performed with painful tediousness. It makes work—hard work—of the act, and that is just as much opposed to Fletcherizing as it is to common sense, horse sense, and all of the natural senses.

Now just for one moment please pay attention to one who is telling you something Mother Nature wants you to know more than anything else in the whole category of intelligence. Fletcherizing is

NOT EXCESSIVE CHEWING

or tedious chewing, or long chewing. The things that require to be chewed long are not good food, and by that sign you may find out their unprofitableness better than in any other way. Good taste from good food is not long lasting. When the mouth is "watering" for the food in sight, or even in thought of it, the coupons of taste they carry with them are short, but represent large figures of satisfaction and nourishment.

MR. GLADSTONE'S ADVICE

Now listen to some figures regarding the number of bites or chews that some foods require under varying circumstances. Mr. Gladstone's advice to his children which has become classic, viz.: "Chew your food thirty-two times at least, so as to give each of your thirty-two teeth a chance at it," was a general recommendation. Mr. Gladstone was observed once when he was a guest at "high table" at Trinity College, Cambridge, and the average number of his "bites" (masticatory movements) as far as they could be counted, was about seventy-five. That did not speak very well for Trinity fare, unless Mr. Gladstone happened to choose food that required that amount of chewing.

Even if Mr. Gladstone did devote seventy-five masticatory movements to each morsel, as an average, such thoroughness would not have involved an unusual length of time for a hearty meal. If you will try the experiment when you are "good and hungry," having a "working-man's appetite," and disposing of good bread and butter the while, which should have nearly, or quite, seventy bites to the ordinary mouthful, you will find that thirty mouthfuls will pretty nearly, or completely, satisfy your working-man's appetite. Mixed foods take much less time, usually about half, and still the seventy-five-rhythm act will consume only about twenty minutes to perform with physiologic thoroughness.

SALIVAL ACTION ON STARCH FOODS

Here are some statements easy to prove or disprove by anyone, with real compensation in the way of new revelations relative to the possibilities of gustatory enjoyment.

Starchy foods, such as bread, potatoes, etc., require from thirty to seventy masticatory movements to assist saliva to turn the starch into "grape sugar," which is the form in which it can be used as nourishment.[1]

You will at once think, no doubt, that a range of numbers extending from thirty to seventy is pretty wide. So it is; but conditions regarding the qualities of not only breads, but potatoes, and also conditions relative to the strength or supply of saliva, differ greatly. When the appetite is keen, the mouth watering, as they are at the beginning of a meal, bread or potatoes may be negotiated into nutriment ready for the stomach in much less time than later on. Appetite "peters," as miners say, gradually, and does not stop with a bang and shut off like an electric light when connection is broken. It checks up, slows down, and tapers off gradually, and that is where the canny intelligence of a faithful Fletcherizer stands himself in good usefulness. When Appetite gently says: "Now, really, you are still rather good to my assistant Taste, and he would not object to a few bites more; but if you stop now and change off to something else which I have in mind, and for which I have a use in our organism, I will not object." In plain words: "I have enough for the present; switch off on to——"

The difference between putting on fat in the case of the person who is disposed or permitted to put on more fat than is comfortable, and losing some of the surplus carried on the abdomen or elsewhere, is the discrimination exercised in regard to the final satisfaction of appetite. Those last two, three, or a few mouthfuls after Appetite has said gently "Enough," and before the same Appetite says, loudly, "Stop!" are the difference between obesity and decency of form.

I really believe, from the results of my experiences for the past fifteen years in getting tips from Mother Nature, and trying to induce mankind in general and my friends in particular to accept them as "straight" from Mother Nature, that persons who have enough respect for themselves to be interested in physical culture must come to the rescue of the pseudo-scientists who are dulled by their own dope, and who are suffering from the malaria which collects in the dark ruts they are following in the tortuous complications of the alimentary canal. The physical culturists must build models of normality for the scientists to study.

When giving information as to what happens in the mouth, and as to what happens as a result of proper head digestion, I feel as if I am sitting on the upper lip of Mother Nature herself, and entrusting her messages to the current of her own sweet breath for distribution among her human children.

CHAPTER VI

WHAT IS HEAD DIGESTION?

My Study of the Subject—The Mouth as a Digestive Organ—Dr. Cannon's Researches—Pawlow's Proofs

In the latest comprehensive treatise on human nutrition, under the title of "Food and the Principles of Dietetics," by Dr. Robert Hutchinson, of London, more than six hundred pages are devoted to the subject. Of these, just fifty lines are given to "Mouth Digestion." In a footnote of sixty-four words Dr. Hutchinson has stated the case of the importance of careful eating, with admission of a fact that would mean emancipation from most of the human disabilities if it were repeated in nurseries and primary schools as religiously as are the ordinary rules of "polite conduct," and held by Society to be the basis of respectability, which it really is.

When I first took up the study of dietetics in academic circles, nearly fifteen years ago, physiologists did not concede that there was any mouth digestion at all. Putting food in the mouth was for the purpose of mixing it with saliva so that it could be formed into a "bolus" for convenient swallowing. Now it is recognised that there is some mouth digestion. In the meantime Pawlow[1] has demonstrated that the psychic influence has much to do with digestion. Cannon, also, has shown by the evidence of the Röntgen rays that mental states retard and even stop entirely the digestive processes that are going on in the stomach, and has asserted, as has also Pawlow, that the stomach digestive juices flow in response to the reports and stimulation of taste, pouring out into the cavity of the stomach juices appropriate for the digestion of the particular food being tasted, in advance of its arrival in the stomach.

This evidence, confirming my own secured by concentrated and unremitting study of the effect of head digestion on health and recuperative reconstruction, is proof enough that there is an important department of nutrition that can be properly called head digestion.

MY STUDY OF THE SUBJECT

began with the tip from Mother Logic—that the full extent of the personal responsibility in nutrition is located in the head before the food is swallowed. That is what led me to concentrate on the mouth as the field of our responsibility which had been neglected by Science. Even the Dental Profession as a whole had not at that time "tumbled" to the fact that they were occupied professionally and constantly in a field of "Preventive Medicine" as important as now they find it.

Everybody had supposed that the digestion of food was effected only in the stomach and small intestines. This may be true, in a narrow sense, but it can be arrested and completely stopped by the head. Furthermore, digestion can be as much assisted by favourable head influence as it can be obstructed by unfavourable head treatment.

This being so, as everybody knows, or can easily learn, what follows as a logical sequence?

Here is a physiological eye-opener, as it dawns upon the business physiologist. The obvious inference is that if the head can make digestion easy or stop it altogether, the stomach being a subservient, mechanical, and chemical servant of the head in the matter, we may properly declare that the master-key of digestion is held by the head, and we may safely say that there is Head Digestion.

THE MOUTH AS A DIGESTIVE ORGAN

The logical continuation of the search for the location of responsibility for good or poor digestion leads us to consider the question of "Division of Labour" as apportioned by the Laws of Normality. All the laboratory evidence I have seen confirms my own observations of the past fifteen years that Nature assures good results if we are thoroughly faithful to our head responsibility during the treatment of food up to the point of swallowing. From that time digestion has been rendered so easy by thorough mouth preparation that it may proceed smoothly even if the mental states are not pleasant. Here, too, we discover that easy digestion reacts favourably on the mentality and exerts a calming influence.

Some observers declare that idiots digest their food quite easily. The less mental clarity they possess the better for their metabolism. This does not argue in favour of the absence of mental influence, for the idiot is a sensualist, and in the relief from mental excitement finds enjoyment of taste and the satisfaction of appetite as agreeable as do the animals under similar favourable conditions.

Quite recently, when I was personally under observation by Dr. Professor Zuntz in Berlin, to test the ease of my digestion of food as compared with others who paid less attention to mouth treatment of it, the good professor instructed me to "be as nearly like a little animal as possible, thinking nothing of anything." This isn't as easy for a "live-wire thinking outfit" as for an idiot, or as for an ingenuous little animal having no thought for the morrow, but the business physiologist does not scorn to go anywhere for light on Nature's requirements. One thing is sure, the person who has been faithful to his personal responsibility by starting the process of digestion as Nature demands can relax and enjoy metabolic and mental calm in delightful harmony more easily than one who has gluttony on his conscience and the wages of sinning on his stomach. These wages look big to the swollen greed of cultivated gluttony, but they are as bad as they are big, and the best way to be convinced of this fundamentally important fact is to realise the potency of head digestion for well or ill, and give it a practical trial.

The key to good digestion is in the head, and the sooner mankind comes to realise this important truth the quicker will come the millennium of nutrition normality.

DR. CANNON'S RESEARCHES

I have just been reading Professor Walter B. Cannon's book in the Arnold Medical Monograph Series, entitled "The Mechanical Factors of Digestion." I have learned many valuable lessons from the intestinal observations of Dr. Cannon, and have seen the shadows he describes on his fluorescent screen under his practised guidance, and, with his generous permission, quoted him extensively in my book, *The A. B.—Z. of Our Own Nutrition.*

It seems that we began our quest for light on the mechanics and mentality of digestion by objective observation about the same year, 1898. He took a hop, skip and jump over the three inches of the alimentary canal that is our personal responsibility and, with the aid of bismuth blackened food and a Röntgen-ray apparatus, began to study the movements incident to digestion by the shadows cast on the screen. For this purpose he principally used female cats, because they were more amenable than male cats to the torture of being tied flat to a cloth with the possible fear that they were condemned to death as well as to inactivity. Even the use of pink or blue ribbons as bands of bondage under the circumstances does not lure their cat-ladyships into the quietude demanded for normal movements of digestion, and male cats will not "stand for it" at all.

For ten years or more Professor Cannon and his assistants were devoted to these Dark Chamber X-ray observations, and in the meantime wading through hundreds of volumes of *Physiological Archives* for reports of other intestinal investigations. The fruit of this thoroughness of research is more than 400 references to reported data and conclusions extending back to the dawn of Physiology. To one who has followed the accounts of the "Diddings" in the "Old Man Greenlaw's Liquor Saloon in Arkansas City," as given weekly in the New York *Sunday Sun*, these researches seem to be governed by the strict rules of "Draw Poker." Eventually all of the cards (or evidence) go into the "discard," confirming Sir Michael Foster's dictum, to the effect that "the more we learn of Physiology the more we know how little we really know."

I recommend everybody to get Dr. Cannon's book and turn at once to page 74, and read about the importance of mastication in securing easy digestion free from fermentation. Then turn to page 217 and read his conclusions relative to the influence of the emotions on digestion. Put these two statements together, and then judge for yourself if it is claiming too much to say that there is really Head Digestion, and that it is in the field of personal responsibility, in the mouth and in the brain, that good or bad digestion—right or mal-nutrition—are inaugurated.

You will find the literary quality of Dr. Cannon's book so fascinating, no matter whether you know the meaning of the terms used or not, that you will enjoy it like a novel. It has the charm of the diction of Sir Michael Foster and Sherlock Holmes combined, with enough of the solving of the secrets of the alimentary canal to satisfy the most exacting imagination.

If a taste for the inner mysteries has been acquired by the reading of Professor Cannon's book, further desires in that direction may be satisfied by reading the physiological prose poem by Professor Chittenden, in praise of head digestion as the acme of sensual pleasure. It is a gem, and is quoted in Chapter VII following, in support of the contention of this chapter. This poem appears in the book *The Nutrition of Man* (as studied mainly in starving dogs), and one wonders why such a pearl of practical, every-day, Kindergarten, domestic usefulness should be "thrown to the dogs," so to speak.

CHAPTER VII

CHITTENDEN ON CAREFUL CHEWING

A Physiological Prose Poem

It is difficult to imagine a more pleasurable Epicurean felicity than that described by Professor Russell H. Chittenden, of the Sheffield Scientific School, of Yale University, in America, as the result of careful masticating and thorough tasting of the commonest of foods.

Professor Henry Pickering Bowditch, of Harvard University Medical School, like Sir Michael Foster and all the most eminent physiologists, were quick to appreciate the revelations of the Cambridge investigation of Fletcherizing as indicating the discovery of the missing link in the chain of processes necessary for securing good digestion and healthy nutrition, but they looked on it as a question of profitable economy rather than material for poetic enthusiasm.

It was given to Professor Chittenden to discover the rarest merit of decent eating; the politeness of it, as well as the poetry; that element of respectability which will eventually recommend it to the socially-refined as one of the civilised fine arts; that expression of appreciation which is due to Mother Nature for her many beneficences.

THE POETRY OF EATING

By Russell H. Chittenden

"With the mind in a state of pleasurable anticipation, with freedom from care and worry, which are liable to act as deterrents to free secretion, and with the food in a form which appeals to the eye as well as to the olfactories, its thorough mastication calls forth and prolongs vigorous salivary secretion, with which the food becomes intimately intermingled. Salivary digestion is thus at once incited, and the starch very quickly commences to undergo the characteristic change in soluble products. As mouthful follows mouthful, deglutition alternates with mastication, and the mixture passes into the stomach, where salivary digestion can continue for a limited time only, until the secretion of gastric juice eventually establishes in the stomach-contents a distinct acid reaction, when salivary digestion ceases through destruction of the starch-converting enzyme. Need we comment, in view of the natural brevity of this process, upon the desirability for purely physiological reasons of prolonging within reasonable limits the interval of time the food and saliva are commingled in the mouth cavity? It seems obvious, in view of the relatively large bulk of starch-containing foods consumed daily, that habits of thorough mastication should be fostered, with the purpose of increasing greatly the digestion of starch in the very gateway of the alimentary tract. It is true that in the small intestines there comes later another opportunity for the digestion of starch; but it is unphysiological, as it is undesirable, for various reasons, not to take full advantage of the first opportunity which Nature gives for the preparation of this important foodstuff for further utilisation. Further, thorough mastication, by a fine comminution of the food particles, is a material aid in the digestion which is to take place in the stomach and intestines. Under normal conditions, therefore, and with proper observance of physiological good sense, a large portion of the ingested starchy foods can be made ready for speedy absorption and consequent utilisation through the agency of salivary digestion.

"Nowhere in the body do we find a more forcible illustration of economical method in physiological processes than in the mechanics of gastric secretion. Years ago it was thought that the flow of gastric juice was due mainly to mechanical stimulation of the gastric glands by contact of the food material with the lining membrane of the stomach. This, however, is not the case, as Pawlow has clearly shown, and it is now understood that the flow of gastric juice is started by impulses which have their origin in the mouth and nostrils; the sensations of eating, the smell, sight and taste of food serving as physical stimuli, which call forth a secretion from the stomach glands, just as the same stimuli may induce an outpouring of saliva. These sensations, as Pawlow has ascertained, affect secretory centres in the brain, and impulses are thus started which travel downward to the stomach through the vagus nerves, and as a result gastric juice begins to flow. This process, however, is supplemented by other forms of secretion, likewise reflex, which are incited by substances, ready formed in the food, and by substances—products of digestion—which are manufactured from the food in the stomach. Soups, meat juice, and the extractives of meat, likewise dextrin and kindred products, when present in the stomach, are especially active in provoking secretion. When the latter foods have been in the stomach for a time, however, and the proteid material has undergone partial digestion, then absorption of the products so formed calls forth energetic secretion of gastric juice. It is thus seen that there are three ways—all reflex—by which gastric juice is caused to flow into the stomach as a prelude to gastric digestion. Further, it has been shown by Pawlow that there is a relationship between the volume and character of the gastric juice secreted and the amount and composition of the food ingested, thus suggesting a certain adjustment in the direction of physiological economy well worthy of note. A diet of bread, for example, leads to the secretion of a smaller volume of gastric juice than a corresponding weight of meat produces, but the juice secreted under the influence of bread is richer in pepsin and acid, *i.e.*, it has a greater digestive action than the juice produced by meat.

The suggestion is that gastric juice assumes different degrees of concentration, with different proportions of acid and pepsin, to meet the varying requirements of a changing dietary."

CHAPTER VIII

THE THREE INCHES OF PERSONAL RESPONSIBILITY

The Effect of Prejudice—Professor Fisher's Experiment

While Professor Cannon was groping about in Nature's alimentary preserves in comparative darkness, I concentrated my attention upon the first three inches of the canal which comprise the field of our personal responsibility, and which has been neglected by most of the students of the subject.

While the area considered was right out in front, and open to visual inspection all the time, the opportunity to study its most important features having to do with nutrition was not continuous. Mr. Edison may rivet his attention on an electrical problem and stick to it for forty-eight hours on a stretch, but Taste is only occasionally on exhibition for observation and cannot be pressed into long service at any one time. For test of normal Taste only the time required for the most economic nutrition is available. A real body-need with keen appetite is the first healthy excuse for calling on Taste to perform. Normal appetite, too, being satisfied with appetising foods, is of brief duration. One may linger over a meal as long as desired, enjoying the intimate memory of the gustatory gratification in leisurely process, but in case of a first-class labouring man's hunger and the exigency of a railway station dinner in the midst of a desert, industrious application of faithful Fletcherizing for fifteen minutes will usually supply the real needs of the moment for eight hours at least. This estimate involves a healthy condition of the nutrition department, including an abundance of powerful saliva for the hastening of the mouth treatment, but such a beatific facility can be secured in a very short time by the faithful and intelligent employment of all departments of head digestion.

A person who specialises on the mouth end of the alimentary canal has plenty of time to rest between inspections. He will naturally watch for any feeling of results that may happen while Mother Nature is doing her twenty-five feet of digestion and absorption, but if his part has been performed properly, there will be no news of the process until there is something to excrete from the material ingested. When this occurs, if a microscope is handy for minute inspection, it will be found that most of the excreta is composed of what I think of as the dandruff of the alimentary canal. It is composed of shapeless particles of skin which have been discarded by the mucous surface of the canal in the same manner that dead skin is being continually detached from the head and all parts of the external surface of the body. Depending on the nature of the food, there may be small particles also of indigestible cellulose from vegetable foods and the condensed solids of the digestive juices when they have been used and worn out.

THE EFFECT OF PREJUDICE

I have noticed that the early prejudices in favour of or against foods are likely to prevail throughout life. I have observed this in trying to secure local appreciation for my own favourite New England dishes in foreign countries. Tinning, or canning, science has made it possible to serve Boston baked beans and brown bread or even an entire Thanksgiving Dinner in Japan or Borneo, but it is impossible to excite native appreciation for them commensurate with the cost and trouble of the transportation. In Scandinavia, where they file the appetite to the keenest of edges with the piquancy of the "Smoer Broed," or "Smoer Goes,"[K] the American taste for very sweet things is not appreciated. Chocolates for that market are more bitter than sweet, and so it goes throughout the world where head digestion is important in determining the prescription of foods.

At one time, during a year and a half of travel in unusual countries where the French, English or American *menu* is not easily available, I never missed an opportunity to study the effect of head prejudice on digestion. If the fortunate opportunity occurs to sample the sumptuous "ris tavel" of Java, there will be the best of chances to confirm my observation in this regard. This dish is varied in sumptuousness, or variety, but the humblest offering of it consists of a large and deep soup plate piled high in the middle with snowy rice with each individual grain unbroken. This, to begin with, is a triumph of oriental culinary art. Surrounding this rice mountain are dabs of every sort of a "relish" any one ever imagined. You select these from tiers of plates borne in each hand by as many as a dozen servants, following each other in procession, and presenting opportunities of choice amounting to twenty or more, perhaps even thirty or more in extraordinary cases. Hence it is the privilege of the guest to take much or little of any, or all, of the condiments according to the state of his appetite or greed. All the colours and nearly the whole food kingdom are represented, and the temptation is increased by the art of rearrangement. There is no way of judging what each sort of relish is: It may be fish, fowl, vegetable, tuber, side-meat, or a combination of nuts or fruits, as far as the intelligence of the uninitiated goes.

There were several members of the party of foreigners of different degrees of prejudice against anything strange in appearance. To one, all of the comestibles were "utterly impossible," and remained so to the end; while to others curiosity got the better of suspicion, and finally the appetites looked forward to dinner-time with especial cordiality, for the rice-mountain relish-cordon and the complicated combination were digested with ease.

The standard dish, however, of the Javan dinner is boiled potatoes and beefsteak swimming in a pint of good butter gravy, so that even the conscientious dietist with vegetarian preferences may revel in something that smacks of home and mother, with such an abundance of luscious fruits that nothing but gustatory delight happens as a usual thing. Still, it is the same in Java or Japan, in London, Paris, Berlin, Vienna, Rome or New York, the digestion of food is under the control of the head and therefore may be called head digestion.

PROFESSOR FISHER'S EXPERIMENT

The most important large experiment for the testing of head digestion under conditions of strict scientific control was that inaugurated and conducted by Professor Irving Fisher, of Yale University, in America.

Professor Fisher occupies the Chair of Political Economy at Yale, has made extensive researches into the factors that influence the economies or extravagances of living, and is President of the Committee of One Hundred of the American Association for the Advancement of Science on Health.

Professor Fisher's interest in my revelations and tests relative to the potency of head digestion came primarily from a personal test which worked wonders for him in establishing a foundation for good health. He was not satisfied with the later Chittenden experiments, because they substituted academic prescription for natural selection in formulating the rules of the inquiry. Like myself, in conducting the original researches, Professor Fisher realised that the practical value of my discoveries was that no one needed a biological chemist to order his meals for him or tell his appetite what his body needed in the way of food elements.

The Fisher experiment worked with nine healthy undergraduates who were ambitious to take high scholastic honours, and who had little time for athletics or any form of physical exercise, they being types of the average University undergraduate.

A generous table was supplied them with meat and every variety of food that usually composed college fare. The only instructions were that thorough mastication and especial attention to the enjoyment of the food as recommended by me in my books should be faithfully performed. This course was pursued for half a year, and for the rest of the year, in addition to the careful head treatment and enjoyment, preference was to be given to foods known to be low in nitrogen content; but not to the extent of suppressing any distinct call of appetite for them.

In the first half of the experiment the men held their own on about 40 per cent. less food, computed by cost, and increased their strength-endurance ability by something more than 100 per cent., with the added felicity of feeling unusually fit all of the time, entirely escaping the slack or sick spells they had been accustomed to, and improving greatly in their general studentability, that is: power of concentration, memory, mental comfort, profundity of sleep, etc.

During the second half of the experiment still more improvement was secured owing to the readiness of the body to accommodate itself to the wish by favouring the economies.

I have not a copy of the report at hand. It is included in the publications of Yale University about 1905.

While all of the abundance of confirmatory evidence which has accumulated since 1898 is valuable and gratifying, the verdict of the unremitting observation since then is that the problem of nutrition is always a personal one. After fifteen years of devotion to the study of the head-end question, with due attention to the tell-tale excreta and the product expressed in terms of energy and general comfort, I am unable to predict what my body is going to want to-morrow in the way of nutrition supply. I can say with some confidence that if I go on doing as I have been accustomed to doing daily, and no shock of grief or surprise intervenes to upset all calculations, I am likely to find nutritive satisfaction as expressed by appetite among the foods that are commonly agreeable to me.

If I am compelled or impelled to do a great stunt of walking or other unusual exertion, or receive crushing news, all my present predictions may be useless. The body itself, from the hair on the head to each finger or toe-nail will know what it wants and will have given to the caterer Appetite its requisition covering the need. In the meantime each brain cell and all of the bones have not been neglectful of their sustenance requirements, nor have they been backward in letting Appetite know.

It is fortunate that the common needs of digestion may be supplied from a limited range of food varieties. Milk is all-sufficient always for general supply of the nutritive requisites. In the plebeian potato, which has attained to royal rank as the result of the extensive experiments of Dr. Hindhede, of Denmark, in co-operation with Madsen the Faithful, has been found full nourishment for ten months, at least, when supplemented by butter or margarine to furnish the fuel supply. Even in this surprising revelation no academic prescription was infallible. Potatoes differ in nutritive value as much as 50 per cent. Fresh-cooked and well-cooked ones alone fill the bill of sufficiency, and full head-work in assuring easy digestion was made the first rule of the test. For four months I served as a check test-subject and speak from experience.

Nothing is ever accomplished except by a division of labour and on the just division of responsibility depends the success of effort. Nature has given to us the head-end of responsibility.

CHAPTER IX

QUESTION PRESCRIPTION AND PROSCRIPTION

The Protein Enthusiast—Doubting Thomases

The only completely accurate prescriber of nutrition for living creatures is Mother Nature herself, and if she does not *pre*scribe anything by the undoubted approval of appetite she *pro*scribes it.

One of the rules which have governed my quest for optimum human nutrition in the midst of the twentieth century food supply and other conditions, has always been to go to Nature for final advice in the matter.

When I say "*Question* Prescription and Proscription" I mean that the most positive prescribers of food have something in the food line or advice to sell, and they proscribe as positively anything that competes with their commercial product.

My eyes were opened to this possible snare and delusion by a great doctor of medicine,[1] who is also one of the most ardent economists I have ever met—not a miser in any sense, but a religiously philosophical economist. He is almost as righteously indignant against any who use the trust which is placed in them by clients or patients for the selling of high-priced foods as he is at the makers, advertisers, retailers and prescribers of alcohol as a beverage. In his just opinion it is as wicked, or almost as wicked, to advise unprofitable extravagance of any sort as it is to prescribe poison.

To this discriminating philosopher food is the basis of health-wealth, and sacred to its divine usefulness.

The great harm that was done to the world by the academic prescription of excessive protein rations[M] was that it started a vicious circle of extravagances which led as surely to untimely death as murder. The perpetrators of this pernicious prescription were innocent of intention to do harm; in fact, they were full of the most generous of motives in issuing their poisonous advice, and one of the most prominent, at least, paid the penalty by dying miserably of his own fatal ignorance.

I may also say that it is "presumption," advisably, for almost all prescriptions of food which do not have their basis on the natural body calls are presumptuous. Nature knows! If given a chance to show her knowledge Nature prescribes rightly and delivers her message in the form of appetite and the other instincts. She will do this in the midst of the most complicated of artificial food mixtures, as I have reason to know from personal experience, confirmed by many others over and over again.

Therefore I may say more surely than ever, that whatever NATURE PROVIDES and PERMITS as NOURISHMENT I HAVE NO RIGHT TO *PRO*SCRIBE.

THE ONLY *PRE*SCRIPTION

that Honesty approves is the Optimum Economic Nutrition; and my great preceptor, Dr. Hindhede, the ideally honest scientist and doctor, ventures to prescribe only the plainest of foods that are delicious to a true, keen appetite, and cost the least through being in season and so common and easy to grow as to be cheapest.

This good and superlatively honest doctor does not *Pro*scribe anything that Nature permits as food and he does not even *Pro*scribe the transportation of grapes from Madeira to the North Cape of Norway for the enjoyment of those who can afford to pay for them.

Would the *Pro*scribers of flesh food have denied Amundsen and his companions the flesh of their faithful dogs as a last resort in securing nourishment for the completion of their journey to the South Pole? It was their truly last resort in gaining the victory over the Ice God; and would to God that brave Captain Scott and his band of faithful ones had had such a last but saving resort to help them accomplish the eleven miles between them and rescue! But then, the world would have missed a model of altruism that is worth a million lives, and one of which million everybody would like to be, if their lives are worth the living.

THE PROTEIN ENTHUSIAST

While writing this chapter I have been forwarded material for indignation and a text for condemnation in the form of a book so full of food prescription that it is positively poisonous, as read with the intelligence of my own and current knowledge of the subject, that it ought to be pilloried as a "Horrible Example" of presumptuous prescription and proscription. It is an advertisement pure and simple, but so prejudicial to the natural facts in the case that it again raises the question of the advisability of a Supreme Court of the Physiology of Nutrition, to try such nutrition perverters for high treason to Mother Nature.

I will not name the book or the author, to further the advertisement. I once stopped a controversy with the doctor-father of the author by offering to wager him one hundred pounds that I could beat him out on a ten mile go-as-you-please tramp, which he had mentioned as one of his stunts to prove his contentions. Our ages were nearly equal, and the difference of training consisted of his prescribing for himself over 100 grams of proteid daily (less by 20 per cent. than the vicious Voit[N] or Kœnig Standards, and less by 30 per cent. than the Standard that killed poor Professor Atwater), while I had subsisted for years on less than half his prescription. He warned me that I was courting death, but that he was providing for himself longevity by the mile. He got mad with me, and nearly fumed at the mouth, because I assumed to insist that only Mother Nature was a competent prescriber, intimating that he was not. I could not out-talk him, and so I sent him a challenge. He made the excuse that he was leaving for the Continent for a rest, but would talk further with me when he returned. His reputed forty-thousand-pound office practice of prescribing his favourite dietaries had worn him out and he was going for a rest. Later I heard of him in a sanatorium—surely disgraceful to a doctor to be compelled to go to such a place for "treatment."

The race, or contest, never took place, but since then I personally have several times broken records established by men one-half, and even one-third, of my age with progressive ease up to three years ago when last put to a test, and I have noted no letting-up of the progress of recuperation as judged by "feelings" or endurance when doing unusual stunts.

In this direction I now feel that I have done enough, and that it is not for age to tempt Providence by competing with the Prime of Muscularity in feats of strength and endurance. John L. Sullivan and Jeffries and many more went once too often into the ring, and Mother Nature, not Corbett or Jack Johnson, knocked them out for good and all. Fletcherizing does not include either imprudence or bluff. It merely trusts good Mother Nature for directions to accompany her nutriment-medicine. Whenever at any time I feel the impulse to turn somersaults from the lead platform of a man-of-war into good, clean salt-water—as I did a few years ago or so in the Philippines, as a demonstration to impress the natives—I will "up and do it, or die in the attempt." What I am doing now more than ever is keeping my ear to the mouth of Mother Nature, my finger on her pulse of command, and doing her biddings as well as I can interpret them. If a thing is not agreeable to do, I take it as a warning *not* to do it. There are so many useful things to do that are pleasant, what is the use of going out of the way to do disagreeable things. There are some things that are natural and agreeable that we should do, and which we have got out of the habit of doing, physical exercise, for instance. We are dealing with cultivated abnormalities always in a cramped and complex civilisation. "We are constantly doing the things that we should not do, and leaving undone those things that we ought to do," as the Prayer Book tells us, including carelessness of eating, and shirking physical exercise.

To return to the callow book of the canny doctor-son of my antagonist of a dozen years ago. It isn't so callow as it is canny, and since the persons in the case are of the canniest of peoples, those who are so shrewd that Jewish merchants do not thrive among them, and the prescription results in thousands of pounds a year revenue, the game may be set down to ordinary commercial cupidity and popular gullibility. It is safe to always warn against Prescription for Revenue. Like patriotism or religion for revenue, it is questionable, if not surely selfishly prejudiced.

On the other hand, Mother Nature charges no fee for her advice. She pays good coin as a premium for her patients in the same way that I bribed my first test subjects into eating right by paying them for eating in addition to furnishing the food.

DOUBTING THOMASES

who are too lazy, or incredulous, or careless, to take a month to try the Mother Nature Prescription as interpreted by me, are liable to say: "Appetite is abnormal. Taste is perverted, and the demands of the body are wholly unnatural."

True! But abnormality of that sort can be corrected in a very short time. A "poor chap" who is lucky enough to have to go without food long enough to "whinney like a horse" at the smell of fresh-baked bread and the thought of good Danish butter on it, is not going to "turn up his nose" at even a crisp baked potato; neither is he likely to require sweetbreads to coax himself to eat. Correcting perverted appetite is like purifying a stream which is being polluted at its source and runs muddy all the way to the sea. Stop the pollution, and the stream will purify itself as fast as ever it can by hurrying along with its impurities to the great ocean sewerage.

CHAPTER X

WHAT CONSTITUTES A FLETCHERITE

Fletcherism and Longevity—W. E. Gladstone, Fletcherite—Fletcherizing Liquids—Getting the Best out of Everything—The Study of Mother-Nature

Since the term "Fletcherite" is incorporated in some of the latest dictionaries, it is proper that the person whose name has been used for the designation should define what constitutes a Fletcherite.

Any person who eats in a healthy manner is a Fletcherite.

Any person who eats in a polite manner is a Fletcherite.

Any person who is faithful to his end of responsibility in securing healthy nutrition for himself is a respectable eater and a good Fletcherite.

WHAT IS NOT A FLETCHERITE

The above definitions are fully comprehensive, but sometimes it is more effective to describe a thing by telling what it is not, and leaving the remainder as an inferential description.

Following this suggestion, it is safe to say, that:

Any one who eats when he is not hungry or what his appetite does not approve, is not a Fletcherite.

All this presupposes the ordinary opportunity for selection in civilized communities where this book is liable to be read and where its revelations and recommendations are most needed.

Any one who does not give his appetite a chance to guide him to healthy nutrition is not a Fletcherite.

Any one who does not extract all of the taste from his food, while it is in the region where taste is developed, is not a Fletcherite.

Any one who succumbs to greed of "getting the worth of his money," because he has paid for food, or can get food free of cost, or takes it on the insistence of Aggressive Hospitality, or to kill time, or for any purpose other than for the satisfaction of a real appetite, is not a Fletcherite.

FLETCHERISM AND LONGEVITY

Returning to positive definition of a Fletcherite: it is a good safe betting proposition that all persons who have passed the seventy year-mark in the life race are Fletcherites in the fundamental requirement of healthy eating. If they reach beyond the eighty year-mark it is certain that they have been fairly decent eaters for many years, even if they abused themselves earlier in life. For example: *vide* the autobiography of Luigi Cornaro, which was concluded only when he was nearly one hundred years old. *Vide* also, occasional newspaper statements attributed to centenarians or near centenarians who claim to have been Fletcherites before Fletcher was born. Some of them have had the "constitution" necessary to attain the respectable longevity and have used tobacco and alcohol at the same time, but there is no evidence that either tobacco or alcohol lengthened their lives. In the same category of questionably-profitable indulgences may be put any of the stimulants or narcotics which do not actually nourish the body.

W. E. GLADSTONE—FLETCHERITE

The Epicureans, who were true to the principles of Epicurus, were Fletcherites, before the name of Fletcher had evolved the occupation of arrow making and archery. Mr. Gladstone was a philosophical Fletcherite before Fletcher discovered that he had a mouth that was worth while studying and using, but the name did not get into the dictionary as describing his most statesman-like inspiration.

A Fletcherite does not confine his Fletcherizing to food. He is encouraged, by the beneficial results of careful eating, to try the same method of co-operating with Opportunity on anything that has good and bad possibilities in it.

FLETCHERIZING LIQUIDS

For example: careful tasting of food reveals felicities of taste which lead to seeking similar rewards wherever taste is to be found. Take liquids: The only liquid that does not invite Fletcherizing with some deliberation, but seems eager to get into the blood to quench thirst is Water. If it is not pure water, soft, cool as if from a spring, and delicious in its purity, it has an inclination to stop a little in the mouth and give taste a chance to investigate or to get something worth while out of it. Do not think that inanimate things have no sense of propriety! Everything natural is as full of propriety as an "egg is full of meat." Nature is Propriety!

Mineral waters, lemonade, beer, wine, and even milk have delicate senses of propriety. They do not rush to be sucked up for the mere relief of thirst, like pure water, but they linger a bit in the domain of taste and inferentially say: "I am tasty;

don't you want to taste me: When I am swallowed my gustatory charm is dead and gone forever; please let me leave my taste with you, good Mr. Taste."

Do not think this is a fanciful personification of the liquids which have taste. Don't take my word for it. I am only telling you what Taste has told me, and also told me to tell it to you. The next time you are thirsty and have a chance to get good pure water, note if it doesn't rush to swallow itself in about one-ounce swallows until the thirst is satisfied. If it is too cold it will want to wait a minute to get to the temperature of the body in the hot room of the mouth, before rushing in to chill the stomach, and if it is too warm it will not give the full satisfaction that spring-cool water gives, showing that Taste has a wider usefulness than mere glorifying of sapid substances. Or: is it Feeling that assists Taste in expressing approval or disapproval of liquid as well as solid nutriment?

GETTING THE BEST OUT OF EVERYTHING

From Fletcherizing things which pass through the laboratory of the mouth, it is most natural to call on Mother Nature in her stately propriety to assist in getting the best and most out of everything from a kernel of corn to the World at Large.

In the personal equipment, muscular exercise, mental discipline, and habits of effectiveness come in at once for analysis and separation.

Outside the personality, companionship is of most vital concern, and the wonder will be how soon the Natural Appetite for profitable companionship will choose some dogs in preference to some human beings, for the qualities of sympathy, approval and faithfulness that every social being craves.

Of course, there are some companionable combinations among men that are more satisfactory and profitable than any dumb animal can possibly supply, but it is for the purpose of finding such combinations that the Fletcherizing of friends is useful. There is much good in every one, as there is in everything that Nature offers as nourishment for the body, but everything has its Appropriate place and time, its harmonious supplements and compliments, and this is true regarding companionships. "What is one man's food, is another man's poison," is a truism applicable alike to companionship and friendship. It is equally true regarding honesty and dishonesty; truth and deceit.

THE STUDY OF MOTHER NATURE

The foregoing constitutes a pretty stiff proposition for the measurement of ideal Fletcherism, but when you come to consider that the aim is nothing less than getting as close to Mother Nature as possible and listening to her orders relative to good team-work between us, the contract does not seem so impossible. It was close study of Mother Nature and her laws of gravity and resistance that led Lilienthal, the German, to try to glide on the "wings of the wind" with imitations of the wings of birds, and it was following Chanute's lead that led the Wright Brothers to develop the flying-machine. It was because of tutelage in the honest school of Mother Nature that the Wright Brothers prefaced their first account of their "invention" by giving the French aviator credit for the initial suggestion.

In similar manner, it was the close, objective study of the psychology of digestion under the honest direction of Mother Nature in a somewhat drastic form that led Pawlow, the Russian physiologist, to preface his account of his great achievement by calling up the memory of the French physiologist Blondlot, and telling that he had described the true process of digestion from logical deduction fifty years before.

In like manner, Professor Cannon, of Harvard University Medical School, insisted that dear Dr. Bowditch, his preceptor in Physiology, had laid out for him the line of X-ray studies of the "Mechanism of Digestion," which has given him distinguished research fame. Getting close to Mother Nature opens up infinite possibilities of enlightenment, and among them cultivation of the honesty and unselfishness which she herself typifies.

CHAPTER XI

ALL DECENT EATERS ARE FLETCHERITES

Dietetic Righteousness—The Disgrace of Sickness—The Optimism of the Fletcherite

In order that there shall be no misunderstanding let us agree upon the dictionary definition of "Decent." It is "Having propriety of conduct."

Let us also take the dictionary definition of Fletcherite, as an agreed meaning. It is: "One who practises Fletcherism."

Fletcherism, in turn, is defined as "A method of thorough mastication recommended by Horace Fletcher."

No self-respecting person wishes to be indecent about anything, and especially about things that are sacred.

I use the term "Indecent" because it has an ugly look and sound. It is more than thoughtless or careless. It is positively indecent and nothing less. So is ugly and irreverential eating more culpable than mere heedlessness when we come to consider what it means in the way of consequences. It spells Indecency from the beginning to the end of the process involved in the act.

You may have a very poor opinion of the namesake in the case, but you must be glad that he discovered for himself that decent eating means recuperation of health if it has been shaken: preservation of health if it is a fortunate possession: and epicurean enjoyment that cannot be realized in full without it.

I repeat that the term Fletcherite is not a personal monopoly but a popular and dictionary creation. I am selfish enough to be glad that Gladstone escaped the distinction of having his great name used as a designation of decent eating.

DIETETIC RIGHTEOUSNESS

When I was called upon to deliver an address before the New York Academy of Medicine on "Possibilities of Recuperation after Fifty," I used a phrase of my own coining, "Dietetic Righteousness," and was later called to account for having been irreverent in using sacred terms in connection with food and eating. "By George!" I replied, in righteous indignation, "Is there anything more sacred than serving faithfully at the altar of our Holy Efficiency?" "Is there any righteousness more respectable than that which furnishes fuel for healthy efficiency and moral stability?" And the question may now be repeated, "Is there?"

As for indecency: Is there any conduct having less propriety than regarding our wonderful mouth, with its prodigious potency for protection and pleasure, as a mere food and drink hopper for good material, which becomes really swill in the alimentary canal if it is not properly treated in the mouth? Can any one think of anything more indecent than offensive odours which are the inevitable tell-tale of indecent eating, and which are eliminated from possibility of development if eating has been decently performed? The penance, or even pleasure, of frequent bathing, in order that the tell-tales of indecency may not become public, does not atone for the sinning in the beginning. The real damage has been done in the, and to the, delicate alimentary canal, with consequences to be realized later on in terms of odious disease or premature death. These are the inside facts in the case made bare by frank presentation.

THE DISGRACE OF SICKNESS

I believe it was the great American philosopher, Emerson, who said that it is "A greater disgrace to be sick than to be in the penitentiary. When you are arrested it is because you have broken a man-made statute, but when you are ill, it is because you have disobeyed one of God's laws." As elsewhere remarked, it is almost impossible in civilized surroundings not to disobey some of the natural laws: body-ventilation, first of all; but no sinning is so dreadfully punished as indecent eating persistently practised.

Some of the ancients believed that the mysterious Something that they called the Soul was located in the stomach and not in the heart or brain. There was reason for thus placing the location, because the bad effect of unhappy thought or anything that "touches the heart" is first felt in the stomach if it has any troubles of its own at the moment to worry about, due to indecent haste or carelessness in eating. To the habitual Fletcherite such double disaster does not come. Easy digestion has been assured by beginning it in the manner required by Mother Nature, and to arrest it by unfavourable psychic influence for a little time does not result in the production of those poisons which wear out the body faster than any other cause. The worst of news may be sprung on one as a terrible surprise, and cloud the happiness for a time without causing damage to the delicate vital organs. Thus the misfortune, or its opposite in disguise, as the case may be, does not set up a vicious circle of accumulating fad effects. The thorough Fletcherite is a philosopher, with a solid foundation for his or her faith in the Good that may be lodged in even seeming misfortune, and the recovery from the shock of disappointment, in order to discover the Good at next hand, is as speedy as desired. The faithful one is ever ready to go before the bar of Death's Tribunal for the approving judgment his dietetic righteousness is sure to secure. Good circles of healthy cause and effect have been swirling about in the organism as the result of faithful decent eating, and Nature or Nature's God never fail to perpetuate the evolution of the Good.

THE OPTIMISM OF THE FLETCHERITE

Fairness or politeness to the part of the wonderful alimentary canal which Mother Nature has assigned to herself to manage is nothing more than common decency; and no privacy of privilege can ever excuse any indecent eating. Just think of all the latitude Mother Nature has given her favourite child man in the way of easy convenience in doing the right thing in eating. He is not compelled to eat every few minutes to keep himself alive, as he is compelled to do in breathing: or every few days, as in hydrating his internal economy with moisture. Never is he caught with his bunkers empty of food for fuel or repair material. Be he as thin as a hatpin, comparatively, he has stored under his skin enough nourishment to last him comfortably for a month. Neither is he terrorised by the conventional gnawing of hunger. He is *per force* wise as to the physiology of nourishment and his stored resources within, and turns any impatience for his habitual rhythm of feeding into a savings bank fund for use when convenient. He is not frightened to death, as indecent thinkers or eaters are, by the prospect of a fast lasting a few hours or days. He knows that he has on him and in him enough reserve supply of nourishment in the form of visible or interstitial fat, and other necessary supply, to last for a long time, forty or fifty days, at least, and there is plenty of time for expected or unexpected relief to happen. He comes to know the value of his mechanism, and the mental and soul essence it produces and supports. His knowledge of his own resourcefulness is sufficient to enable him to conserve all vital strength until hoped for relief comes. Or, being in tune with the good intentions of the Universal Life of which he is a part, he never dreads the promotion we call death. It is merely a station on the road of evolution, and just as sure as we are of death and taxes, so is a faithful Fletcherite certain that he is travelling the road of natural evolution. He has not only eaten decently in the way of fulfilling the natural mechanical and chemical requirements in the mouth, but he has abstained from eating when the mental state was not favourable, and has refrained from worry when the prospect of a meal was deferred for a little while or indefinitely. He may have been whinnying like a healthy horse in anticipation of revelling in the delights of delicious taste, and yet is not filled with disappointment at the postponement of the expected pleasure if the dinner appointment is upset or delayed.

This quite Utopian possibility of stable equanimity is the assured result of consistent decent eating, and thinking relative to nutrition. It is the constitution and bye-laws of Fletcherism.

As a natural presumption, when decency in one direction leads to such delightful fruition, the opposite of it, indecency, must swing its pendulum to the extent of its full scope in the contrary direction, and it does, for compensation is one of the laws of Nature that must be fulfilled. It is true that Nature is always trying to accommodate herself to any abuse. She may permit being so much accustomed to it that the punishment of it at the moment is not noticed. She even encourages the acceleration of the vicious circle that leads to momentary bankruptcy of resistance, penitence, and reform, as in the case of "bilious attacks." The man who takes his daily or hourly prescription of alcoholic stimulant is permitted to believe that if a little seems good, more should be better until he is landed under the table. He becomes more and more efficient in "standing" the abuse until "under the table" means "under the sod." The abuses have, however, been just as disagreeable to Normality all the way along as the first drop of alcohol was distasteful to the infant in arms. So, too, with tobacco, in a less violent form.

Faithful practice of decent eating reverses the order of progress. Normality of taste is the new direction taken. Appetite is given a chance to discriminate, and it chooses simple food, having the chemical constituents required by the body at the moment. It accommodates itself to the daily activity, and can be trusted as the only completely-wise prescriber of what food to take, and how much of it the body can utilize just then.

Herein lies the value of decent respect for Appetite in securing optimum digestion and nutrition. It does not treat all persons alike because no two persons can be alike. Infinite variety is the fundamental law of Nature. Some persons are born to carry more fat than others. To try to keep them thin is a sin against the natural intention. To allow them to become too fat is also a sin. Strictly decent eating settles this question in conjunction with the sort and amount of activity that the particular person is intended by his or her "Hereditary Tendency" to exert.

CHAPTER XII

FLETCHERIZING AS A TEMPERANCE EXPEDIENT

Tramp Reform—A Remarkable Man—How to Enjoy Wine—Fletcherism as a Cure for Morbid Cravings—A Trial of Fletcherism and its Results—Fletcherism as First Aid

Now we come to a phase of the merits of Fletcherism which has already furnished an abundance of evidence to its credit. In my first experiment, not yet under academic supervision, with no laboratory measurements wherewith to describe the results in chemical terms, I was dealing with a company of ordinary tramps picked up in the streets of Chicago. They simply ate what they chose to order from the bill of fare of a cheap restaurant, but were told to chew everything for all it was worth, which they made no objection to doing. Time was of no value to them, and they really discovered new delights of gustatory pleasure which they had not known before. Tramps are generally persons of resourcefulness and have a cultivated appreciation. Their resourcefulness consists chiefly of being able to live without working, and their appreciation is made keen by the lottery of chance in seeking to get something for which they give nothing.

My tramps were beery and bleery as tramps generally are, but not so dirty; for I paid for baths, washing, and in some instances furnished clothing. Besides supplying these luxuries, I gave them occasionally a big silver dollar which they called a "cart wheel."

It was surprising to see these degenerates freshen up in appearance and lose their blotchiness and greasiness of facial appearance. I knew how to talk to them to get their confidence, and they looked on me as just another "freak" like themselves, but with some kind of a money "pull."

There were fat and thin among them, and it was a matter of surprise that after a little some of the thin got stouter and the fat fell off in weight at the same time. One of them was a belligerent socialist and the author of a well-known book which had quite a vogue in the earlier history of present-day socialism.

Up to the time I began my own experiment, I had been a social drinker of alcohol in all forms to the full extent of "gentlemanly decency," with occasional slips when near the outer edge that made me ashamed of myself after I got sober again. I am now more ashamed than ever when I am reminded of my early foolishness, but since my experiences are being turned to good account I forgive myself. Not only were social occasions an excuse, but I often ordered the social occasions to serve as an excuse. I had never resorted to snake-bites to give legitimate excuses, but I so crowded my resources in this direction that at one time I held the "record," for the community in which I lived, for what was called "hollowness of legs and steadiness of head," and so much was this "strength of character" valued in that community in America, that one was supposed to take pride in holding the record.

The result of my own pursuit of thorough tasting of my food had been that my own ponderosity of front weight fell off, and at the same time I had no desire for wine or beer. It was all a surprise to me, but it was not an amazing surprise until one day one of my tramp guests came to me and said: "Boss, this eatin' game is great; think of me with a dollar in my pocket and not wantin' beer."

In a short time I forgot that I had ever liked wine or beer. It never occurred to me to order it except for a guest, and then I took it with him, or, rather them, for there were usually several or many at my eating parties, but in the Fletcherian manner which is so eminently Epicurean that a few sips went as far as a half-bottle used to do. Here is an important point in profitable economics that any one can demonstrate for himself at once and not rely on my sayso, or that of any one else. Later on I will tell how to do it. The secret is worth its weight in gold as an Epicurean prize as well as a money-saver. I have to tell, a little further on, of a very large experiment which came as a surprise also. It was in a section of country, and among a class of people, where to escape from the toils of the drink demon is nothing short of a miracle.

A REMARKABLE MAN

But before I relate this climaxic experience I will once more refer to one of the most remarkable men I have had the pleasure of meeting. His case covers more sides of healthy variety than that of almost any one, but he has even a better showing in some respects than any. He is an M.D.; a Ph.D.; an Sc.D.; an A.M.; and a P.H.D.; which last is the "stiffest exam." of them all. He is a champion athlete; the father of an all-round college champion; and as graceful a gymnast as any one ever saw do the "Giant Swing" on the horizontal bar. He is also a grandfather and now past fifty.

This was his experience in 1902 or 1903, in connection with my being called to New Haven to submit to examination under the supervision of Professor Chittenden. It is Dr. Anderson to whom I refer, and he permits my stating his experience as often as I like for the good it will do. My expression of appreciation of his academic and athletic accomplishments is all my own and not authorized.

When I was turned over to Dr. Anderson for physical examination in the Yale gymnasium, my fitness was surprising to him as he has stated in his reports. He was also ripe for the reasonableness of my revelations. He seemed to me to be in the "pink of condition" himself, and he was so, as "pink" was judged at the time, for a man of his age.

Dr. Anderson tried more careful mastication than usual, and paid more attention to the thorough enjoyment of his food with the same pleasant results that come to everybody when making the trial, no matter how moderate and temperate they have been before. It is equivalent to putting a little keener edge on appetite than usual. Children and even fine ladies will perk up a little when they are conscious of being noticed, and the human senses are human in more ways than one.

Dr. Anderson was pleased with the revelation as a pleasure promoter, but did not notice that he was forgetting to take his daily prescription of stimulant. He was a medical man, past forty, beginning to slack up a little in his elasticity and strength. He was reaching that age when even the most temperate and careful begin to be a little lenient with themselves. His doctor friends were in the habit of prescribing a little stimulant to counter-balance this expected decline in energy and he took their advice. It was the medical fad of the period.

At first, Dr. Anderson ordered for himself one small drink of good medicinal whisky a day, and the effect was as expected. By and bye, however, a little more was needed, and this increasing demand continued its insistence until three drinks were no more efficacious than one had been at first. When I was introduced to him he had begun on his fourth drink daily, and yet burned it up in his exercise without feeling it much.

A couple of weeks after he began to check up my test by personal experience, which is the only scientific way, he all at once remembered, one day, that he had forgotten to take his whisky, and yet he was fitter than usual. I had not mentioned my own experience in this regard to him, I believe, as when we were together he kept me busy with the exercises of the 'Varsity crew, and I had little chance to give him accounts of my full experience. Besides, it did not occur to me that it would interest him who seemed to be moderation and temperance personified. And so he was, according to the scientific estimate of the time, but Nature has another standard of temperance, and under her strict guidance very little but good spring water is needed or desired.

HOW TO ENJOY WINE

To illustrate this and also suggest a way of letting Mother Nature prove that I represent her correctly in this important matter, I will give an account of an actual happening.

I was lecturing in Buffalo, New York, in America, and was invited to address the members of the sumptuous Buffalo Club. I dwelt especially on Fletcherizing as a means of getting the good and the best out of food and drink, and yet for little cost, and at the close of the lecture a dozen or more of the audience asked me to demonstrate my point as above. I was happy to do this, and called for a pint of the choicest still wine, with cordial glasses. The request caused a smile among some of my hosts who were proud of being "one bottle" consumers.

When the wine came I poured out half a cordial glass as the portion I selected for myself and recommended the same prescription for the others, as a "starter." Then I breathed and sipped my delicious grape-juice, as I had learned to do from the professional wine-tasters on the Rhine, in Germany, and in the Burgundy region, in France. The others did the same, and seemed to get unusual satisfaction from both the *bouquet* and the taste.

What happens is this: You sense the wine by means of the olfactories as you would breathe in the odour of a delicately perfumed flower. Taste is excited and becomes jealous of Smell. You give Taste a taste. Something more subtle than taste; a sort of aroma, so to speak, spreads over the head. You feel the taste of the delicacy up around the temples, and the sensation is delightful in the extreme, fading slowly away but leaving a lovely memory impression.

Then you take another sip, and the sensation is about the same, and so on for a sip or two more, when the supremest delicacy of the wine ceases to express itself. Two or three sips more, and the wine no longer tastes good. Carried further, in this appetite-respecting manner, there will be a desire to spit out the sips, and there is no temptation to drink them.

Professional wine-tasters are supposed never to *drink* wine. After tasting it they spit out the remnant from which the taste has been exhausted. Tea tasters and beer tasters and special food tasters do the same in order to preserve their keen taste discrimination.

There is just as definite Swallowing Sense and Expectorating Sense as there is Taste Sense. There is just as strong Appetite Sense for proteid, when the body is short of it, as there is thirst-demand for water for the rehydration of the body. The Senses have sense!

Returning to the Buffalo Club experiment in demonstrating Epicurean Temperance: The half-bottle of wine gave more satisfaction to the dozen or more members of the Club who participated in the experiment than any of them knew was possible.

FLETCHERISM AS A CURE FOR MORBID CRAVINGS

It is not necessary to supply expensive wine for the complete satisfaction of the most delicate epicureanism if Fletcherizing is employed as an habitual cream-separating means. The cream of common wheat bread, and of anything that the normalized appetite favours, is as satisfying when the body is in need of what it contains as are drops of the most costly Johannisberger of the rarest vintages, and nothing but water thoroughly quenches real thirst.

The "testimonials" of one sort and another, including letters and verbal account, attesting to the effect of natural eating on abnormal desires or cravings, number thousands. The reform has not been the result of suggestion, although in some cases suggestion has assisted the cure of intemperate yearnings. Not alone has craving for alcoholic stimulant been abated, but in other ways morbidity has been corrected, and I as well as some medical men I know, have received grateful acknowledgment of the happiness secured by the natural sloughing off of weaknesses or passions which had been a source of self-hatred. Think what immunity from such baneful possibilities means to youth of both sexes!

A TRIAL OF FLETCHERISM AND ITS RESULTS

The very large test of Fletcherism as a temperance expedient hereinbefore referred to was entirely accidental. It occurred in a community of students of a missionary college in Tennessee.

The institution is conducted under religious auspices, the sect supporting it being that called "Seventh-Day Adventists." The buildings are on a large farm, and most of the students earn their board and tuition by doing farm work. Many subsist by what is called "boarding themselves," that is: purchasing raw food and doing their own cooking. To assist in this independence there is a commissary where everything needed is bartered or sold.

One of the prominent persons in the Adventist denomination is Dr. Kellog, Superintendent of the Battle Creek Sanatorium, who from the beginning has been one of the most ardent advocates and teachers of Fletcherism, and to whom is largely due the permanency of its designation as "Fletcherism."

During a visit to the Tennessee institution, Dr. Kellog so successfully preached the merits of natural eating, that all the students were induced to give it a trial as a health and economic measure.

The trial was conducted under observation for six months, when an accounting was made. During the six months the drafts on the commissary had been a trifle less than half what they formerly had been, and at the same time the community had been free from the usual "seasonable" and bilious complaints or illnesses. No one had been cured of a craving for alcohol, for the reason that all were teetotalers on principle, but the sheer economy and healthfulness of the results obtained were of prodigious importance to young persons "working their way through college." The amount of the benefit can be imagined when it is considered that they needed to work less on the farm to earn their food because the food-bill was much reduced. The time saved from work was available for study, and the increase of energy and immunity from sickness added enormously to the average student ability.

One day there was brought to the institution on a stretcher a poor chap of the neighbourhood, crazy with delirium tremens. In the infirmary of the college emergency patients were received, as part of the missionary training is medical.

The sorry dipsomaniac was sobered-up in the usual way and instructed in the process of Fletcherizing. He took kindly to it, as all do who have been dietetic sinners, and the result was the same as with the beery and bleery tramp mentioned in the early part of this chapter. He lost his "taste" for "booze" and continued the incident by becoming a worker on the place and a sound temperance example.

Here is a revelation worth while to the missionary workers. Their field of service was the mountain districts of their State and the neighbouring State of North Carolina, which are famous for their moonshine whisky stills. The whisky distilled in the mountains does not pay any Internal Revenue tax if it can be avoided, and hence the stills are hidden in deep forests and operated by the light of the moon. The inhabitants of these lawless regions are the poorest of the poor and call down the contempt of the negroes. They are called "poor white trash," and moonshine whisky that will kill at fifty yards is responsible for much of the poverty and trashiness. They are as good marks for missionary sympathy as any "heathen" the world can produce anywhere. I have been among them all and I assure you, these listless and luckless inebriates of the poor white trash regions are the most pitiable.

FLETCHERISM AS FIRST AID

As soon as the incident of the victim of delirium tremens had been measured at its full significance, it dawned upon the missionaries that Fletcherism was to be their most potent assistant in curing the mountaineers of their vices and preparing them for religious instruction. They were won over to the ideal of Dietetic Corpoculture as "First Aid to the Injured" in establishing Temperance on a sound basis.

Thus it was that the graduated missionaries introduced themselves to their charges by building simple ovens of road-side stones in rail-fence corners, as field surveyors might do, and invited those who came along to feed with them.

There is never any trouble in securing guests at a feed anywhere, and it is extremely easy among the poor to whom free food means less work and more leisure. It is easy, too, to get the ears and attention of guests at meals who would like to be invited again. It is also easy to teach Fletcherizing to youthful dinner-guests, as Madame La Marquise de Chamberay and I found out in connection with our East Side investigation in New York.[0]

The result of this strategy on the part of the Tennessee missionaries was reported to a meeting at the Battle Creek Sanatorium, and the summary of the good attained up to that time was as follows: More than a thousand persons were saving an average of $3.00 a month on the cost of their sustenance, and were temperance converts through the sloughing off of all desire for their moonshine product. Think of a saving from sheer waste of $3,000 a month ($36,000 a year) to a community where $1,000 is considered to be a princely fortune, and a saving of a thousand human units from the scrap-heap of worse than death!

CHAPTER XIII

THE MENACE OF MODERN MIXED MENUS

Gluttony and Avoirdupois—Contentment—Fletcherism and Political Economy

While it is true that "Variety is the spice of life," and that an appetising variety of plain food is more tempting than a monotony of the most highly-spiced dishes, every tendency of modern menus is a menace to health, and the only way to counteract the menace is to be especially careful in observing the rules of Epicurean Economy.

If the soup is particularly good, there is a temptation to go on and completely satisfy the appetite on it. It requires the restraint of civilized suppression to keep from following the example of Oliver Twist, calling for more and more till the supply or appetite is exhausted.

Then comes the fish: Who can resist accepting a generous helping of this course, served in any one of the dozens of styles that are familiar to the patrons of French restaurants? And how hard it is to refrain from cleaning up the plate in a hurry so that none of it will be whisked away by the waiter to make room for course number three.

Nothing has been said of the Hors d'œuvres of the French menu, or the Ris Tavel of the Dutch East Indian gorge, or the Smoer Gose of a Scandinavian "Spread." A fairly ravenous person, given time enough, and with no one looking, can be counted on to make a "square meal" on these "appetizers" alone before the soup is announced.

Mention of the "*Roast,*" the "*Entrées,*" the "*Légumes,*" the "*Dessert,*" and a bewildering variety of cheeses to be followed by fruit, nuts and raisins, with several different wines, cordials, coffee, and cigars or cigarettes on the side. Even mention of them is likely to cause psychic indigestion.

If one goes to a restaurant with a quarto, gilt-top appetite, and scans one of the monster, modern, mixed menus for a suggestion of what he shall order, he will, undoubtedly, see five or six items that will appeal to his imagination as "just the thing"; and if the cost is no special reason for restraint, he will put down on his order list twice or three times as much as he can possibly eat in order to be as many kinds of a *fam dool* as he can be at the moment.

This is not an unreasonable or fantastic illustration of the menace of a multiple menu and a colossal appetite in convenient conjunction. It is said that an amorous lover has neither conscience nor discretion. This may sometimes be the case; but it is always a sure betting proposition that an opulent, ravenously-hungry person will measure off with his eager eyes much more than his tummy can possibly hold.

Then follows the inclination of the average human being to "get his money's worth," even if he "must die for it." This is not alone a human characteristic exaggerated in sumptuously-civilized communities, but it is an animal trait as well. If a racehorse is turned out in a field of clover that stands as high as his neck, he will very likely eat himself to death. Likewise, if a little child, with the animal characteristics uppermost, is given a bag of sweets, he will be sure to want to put himself securely outside of the whole bag-full in the shortest time possible, so that he will make certain that no one will take it away from him.

GLUTTONY AND AVOIRDUPOIS

The menace of the munificent menu also leads to the uncomfortable acquisition of surplus avoirdupois. On some persons it has quite the opposite effect, however. The writer remembers that it was a tradition in his college that the thinnest man of a class was always the biggest glutton. Each year, a prize of a combination knife, fork, and spoon, was given to the grossest eater of the junior class. Within my memory the recipient was always a very thin and cadaverous fellow.

As a matter of fact, the hardest work done by the body is performed within the body. It is the work of digestion, general metabolism, and the constant and never-ceasing pumping of the blood through hundreds of miles of veins and arteries. If this work is measured in terms of heat units thrown off (calories) the internal activity of the body is as two to three parts of the whole heat energy released into the surrounding air.

It is quite possible to increase this heat expense by 20 to 50 per cent. by merely overloading the stomach a little, and crowding the mechanism of metabolism to its utmost. Sometimes the crowding is carried so far that the organism cannot stand it; sometimes bursts; and, there you are—dead.

CONTENTMENT

The supremest felicity is not wanting anything. If one cannot think of a single thing in the wide, wide world, not even oblivion, that they would have in addition to what they are enjoying at the moment, their cup of contentment is full.

In regard to eating, to have Fletcherized a few morsels of the finest food that anyone's mother ever made, until there is no desire for more, and yet the contentment is of that calm sort that indicates that there is no overloading of the stomach, is gastronomic Heaven, and it carries with it a blanket of general contentment that covers the universe.

On the other hand, to have eaten unwisely, as the result of animal voracity, over-estimate of capacity, and greed of getting outside of all that must be paid for, or, in slavish deference to aggressive hospitality, is Hell from the finish of the meal until the finish of the "spell of sickness" that may follow the gorge. It were almost possible to sink into the depths of such gluttony on any one, two or three of the best dishes possible to imagine; only a modern multiple mixed menu is liable to bring this degradation, and hence the menace of it.

Suppose, again, you are framing up a business deal, and have a customer "on the string." The best way to get at his heart and pocket-book is through the sociability accompanying a sumptuous meal.

You seek a Princess' Restaurant, a Ritz-Carlton or a Waldorf, and make a spread of your Epicurean generosity, your bank account, and your business web or net. If you insist on filling your guests full of everything, you must set the example. Results: Similar in all cases.

Science is not even secure against the temptation of the monumental menu. The writer has known the citadel of scientific conservatism to be captured by five-dollar still-wine and fifty-cent cigars, as accompaniments of six-course dinner-dreams. This, too, in the interest of an Epicurean Economy that put all of the academic teachings in the back-number list, and favored fifty-cent banquets with nary a cigar to top off the feast.

FLETCHERISM AND POLITICAL ECONOMY

It may be argued that the waste attendant on sumptuous living is the most prolific means of keeping money in circulation: of putting bread into the mouth of the servant class: and that Spartan simplicity would throw the world back two thousand years in the civilized progress it has made.

That might be true of some forms of sumptuousness, but not as to the wanton waste of food through the temptations of magnificent menus. Food is the realest of all forms of wealth. Scarce ever a grain of wheat or kernel of corn is wasted. The story of the Englishman who visited Kansas, and from there took home to London a colossal joke at the expense of corn and Kansas, illustrates the permanence and indestructibility of food wealth.

Riding through the State, with a native Kansan, an English globe-trotter wondered at the endless fields of yellow "maize." He called it maize, but the Kansan called it "corn."

"What in the world do you do with all this maize?" said the mobilized Cockney. "Oh, that is easy," replied the native: "We eat what we can and we *can* what we can't."

In due season this strange answer was interpreted to the visitor and he determined to can the joke for serving up at his club in London.

Arriving in England, the joker made deliberate preparations to open his can of Kansas corn to the best effect. He invited a set of chappies to dine with him and the *pièce de résistance* was Kansas canned corn.

Having engineered the matter to the right point of curiosity, the host told the story of his visit to Kansas and finally exploded his *finale* in this wise: "Do you know, these Americans out in the West are a jolly lot. They have a dry sort of wit, too. I was travelling in company with one of them through the State of Kansas, which is the great maize State of the country. They don't call it maize, however, they call it corn, and what we call corn they call wheat. Well, I was amazed at the miles and miles of maize—no pun intended and no apology needed—and asked my companion whatever in the world they did with it all. And what do you think he said: He said, 'We eat what we can and the rest we put up in tins!'"

It took the perpetrator of the joke another week to find out why no one laughed, and spoiled everything by still waiting for the point after the real explosion took place: and no international incident is recorded in the history of that day.

Yes, the really most vital wealth is stored in the food treasuries. Profusion of it carries down the prices and this raises wages by comparison. There is always a spot-cash market for food at some price, which is not the case with many other forms of property.

But the waste of the food material itself is insignificant compared to the waste of energy that must take place to get rid of it, the moment it is swallowed and beyond personal responsibility. The transportation of a carload of wheat by rail from Saskatchewan to the Atlantic seaboard by rail and across the ocean by steamer is small as compared with the expense of getting a mouthful of bolted bread through an alimentary canal that is congested with indigestion.

CHAPTER XIV

THE CRUX OF FLETCHERISM

The Value of Occasional Fasting—The Power of Freedom from Indigestion—Muscles have Memories

Almost everybody eats with sufficient care most of the time; otherwise, all would be on the sick-list *all* the time and the death-rate would be increased enormously.

Whatever sickness, depression, weakness and other illnesses there are now are the result of occasional carelessness only.

The remedy for lapses from carefulness is knowledge of what the natural requirements are, and training the muscles and functions employed in nutrition to work always with careful deliberation and never allow themselves to be hurried with their work.

It should also be made a habit

NOT TO EAT ANYTHING

without a keen appetite. This involves knowing how to recognise a true appetite and also how to detect a false craving. Waiting for a healthful call for food, for any length of time, can do no harm, and should not cause any discomfort or inconvenience; but exciting a false desire and taking food before the body is "good and ready" for it, starts trouble brewing at once.

If the worst results of premature or hurried eating were immediately felt, no one would get in the habit of sinning in this manner. Like auto-intoxication from excess of alcohol, poisoning from unnecessary or unwelcome food—either an excess of it or when taken untimely—is an aftermath of unhealthy stimulation or exhilaration.

The crux, then, of dietetic righteousness, or, Fletcherism, is habituating the body to practise that Eternal Vigilance, which is

THE PRICE OF FREEDOM FROM INDIGESTION

It should be much easier to instal a habit of carefulness than it is to permit habits of carelessness. It is possible so to sensitize the muscles which control swallowing that they will refuse to act and will cause choking if an attempt to swallow prematurely is made. Systematic attention to this detail of care for a week will secure it as a permanent habit without need of any further attention to it.

The statement that it is easier to do the right thing than it is to do the wrong thing: and that it is easier to fix firmly good habits than it is to acquire bad habits, will probably be questioned or disputed by many; but practice of the principles which underlie Fletcherism will cure such pessimism relative to the attitude of Mother Nature towards her most perfect product in general, Man.

Man is given more liberty and more license than any other natural expression and, with the endowment which we call "intelligence," he is raised to a position of partnership in assisting natural evolution and progress.

From inklings of experience it is reasonably inferred that Man is more susceptible to evolutionary influence than any of the animal kind; that he can ever progressively train himself towards higher and higher supermanhood; that he is able to perform marvels in taming and training other animals and in perfecting plant life to prodigious proportions. He is even "gifted" to the extent of overcoming, harnessing, and using at will the "forces of Nature," and dispelling the mysteries. He can only do this, however, by co-operating with Nature in the most intelligent and faithful manner.

To ascertain Nature's requirements of preferences it is necessary to begin with the first essentials of care, the nutrition of the body and the management of the mind. These basic essentials are the first concern of Fletcherism and really the crux of the Scientific Management of the Highest Efficiency.

One of the most important discoveries in the development of Fletcherism is the fact that

MUSCLES HAVE MEMORIES

The usefulness of this discovery rests in the knowledge that it is possible to make the muscles connected with nutrition commit to memory the sequences of procedure in the processes of nutrition which accomplish the most profitable results, and then pass on to other details of responsibility care-free and thought-free, fully confident that everything will go on as Nature would have it go.

Without beginning this discipline of the muscular equipment at the right point and in the right manner, no solid structure of Efficiency-Building can be secured. Any amount of indigestion, or unnecessary strain put upon metabolism, interferes with the smooth working of the organism in the same way that an infinitesimal weight put at the tip end of the long arm of a lever multiplies the burden of resistance at the short end many, many fold.

Therefore, the Crux of Fletcherism is found in first training the muscular and mental apparatus to proceed with thorough deliberation relative to every thing taken into the body; for from this intake, and especially from the manner of the handling of this material along the line of the alimentary canal, come efficiency or inefficiency.

It is first necessary to know what you want the muscles to habituate themselves to doing in connection with nutrition. They must learn to know what constitutes a true appetite, in contradistinction to indefiniteness of want or desire. The muscles will soon learn to know that real hunger (body need) is not expressed by any uncomfortable feelings below the guillotine line. Only in the head, where the senses are all bunched together for the most important team-work, is honest hunger sensed. We may rightly add to the list of the senses, Appetite, and trust it with confidence to tell us what the body can use to advantage of the foods available at the time. That the foods are appetizing is the only recommendation necessary to a set of muscles trained to treat them as Nature requires when they enter the laboratory of the mouth.

Connected with the training of the mouth-muscle outfit, there is the one standing order. Challenge everything applying for entrance, whether by special invitation or in the way of surprise, by testing it for taste-acceptability at the tip of the tongue. Then keep on tasting and testing, with reverential appreciation of the gustatory delight there is in it, in the full knowledge that both digestion and assimilation, which are the prime necessities of nutrition, are healthfully stimulated by accentuated enjoyment.

It is not necessary to dwell intensively on sensual enjoyment of the material being automatically handled by the methodical muscles. The pleasant sense sensations surrounding taste may serve as an accompaniment to agreeable conversation, to the delight of beauty in any form, to flowers, to music, to graceful and vivacious femininity, or to any sort of charm, with added strength given to the effect on wholesome nutrition.

So much for the usefulness of the mouth-muscles, including that most wonderful of muscles, the tongue, in assisting in the healthful stimulation of nutrition. Their most important office is to stand guard against the contingencies that are liable to happen which are prejudicial to digestion. If there is worry in the atmosphere: "Don't let anything into the mouth on pain of court-martial and suffering!" Those are the "orders of the day" for the sentinel muscles of the mouth, serving at the outer entrance of the alimentary canal.

In the category of "worry" are included anger, argument, blues, or any other of the depressant passions, and no food or drink, other than water, should be admitted to the canal while any form of depressants are being suffered.

We must agree in the first place that it can do no harm to wait for a clearance of the mental atmosphere. Real hunger is not a painful craving for something or anything, but is a most accommodating waiter for final collection of all the taste dividends there are due in a big lump sum to compensate for not getting them by instalments. Consequently, if the mental atmospheric conditions are not favourable to the best nutrition, the best way to clear them is to wait. Nothing is so forceful in making one modify or forget passing clouds of pain or disappointment as growing healthy Hunger.

The mouth-muscles soon learn to know this beautiful provision of Mother Nature, whereby deferred collections by appetite are paid with compound interest sometimes sure, if by the waiting process the mental atmosphere is cleared of the elements of digestive lightning and thunder.

How delightful it is to be assured that the best way to secure the best nutrition is the easiest way and that it can be quickly installed as a habit, so that attention to the mechanics of the care is not necessary, leaving the whole battery of appreciation to employ itself with the gustatory festival.

CHAPTER XV

FLETCHERISM AND VEGETARIANISM

The Danger of Excess of Protein—The Use of Meat and Uric Acid—To Sum Up—Profitable Economy

In the warfare against the "Demons of Dietetic Disturbances" most of the volunteer recruits go into the camp of the *Mealers*, that is, they become vegetarians, *quasi*-vegetarians, or partial vegetarians, and array themselves against human carnivorous habits and practices. They are comparatively few in numbers, but make up in enthusiasm what they lack in numerical strength. Some of them base their objection to meat-eating on physiological grounds, others on sentimental susceptibility, and yet others are influenced by reasons of economy.

With world-wide and centuries-old evidence before me in forming an opinion, I say without hesitation that the weight of argument is in favour of a meatless diet most, if not all, of the time, and that all who subsist on the first-hand fruits of the soil and do not resort to cannibalism, except in cases of emergency, are on the safer side.

THE DANGER OF EXCESS OF PROTEIN

To mention the greatest danger from using meat for nutrition first, we find it almost impossible to eat most meats without taking into the organism more protein (nitrogen) than is required for repair of the broken-down tissues; and we now know that any excess of protein or nitrogen imposed upon the body is not good for it. Large excess is positively deadly in its final effects, and many, if not all of the so-called uric-acid troubles or diseases are traced to such abuse.

Not only are the kidneys worn out long before their time, but high blood-pressure is one of the baleful results that lead to untimely demise. To be sure, persons are reported to have lived to near or quite an hundred years of age as habitual *meat*ers, but their occupations or activities have been favourable to burning up the dregs of metabolism, and the belief is reasonable that if they had not been thus self-abusing during the first century of their life they might have gone quite a piece into the second century with their matured experience, example, and wisdom, serving the world to good advantage.

THE USE OF MEAT

That meat is an emergency expedient in the natural nutrition of man is pretty certain. Strictly speaking, we are all of us subsisting on meat all of the time, but it is only *one degree removed from the vegetable kingdom*, when we ingest only the first fruits of the soil, as vegetarians do, and make meat of it within us. The vegetable nutriment is transformed into our own flesh and blood in the form of fat chiefly, and then is used to furnish whatever heat and repair material we happen to need. When second-hand, already dead and decomposing meat is eaten and thus used for life-giving purposes, it is really not only second-hand supply but third-hand material. For instance, we may subsist exclusively on vegetable or farinaceous material and get our repair or fuel supply from such sources only. The result is, in part, the forming of the walls of our own stomach. These walls are meat. Should we turn into cannibals, devouring each other as the Pacific (?) Islanders used to treat missionaries and enemies, the stomach walls become tripe and are easily digestible. While they were live walls, holding in place glands secreting powerful gastric juice, they resisted the digestive aggression of their own juice, but the moment they were separated from their own living combination, quite similar gastric juice digested them as quickly as it does the white meat of a pet chicken. It is physiologically possible to cut out a part or the whole of our own stomach, and then devour and digest it as tripe in the small intestines.

Hence it is that we are all *meat*ers, perforce, but not all of us are third-degree-removed cannibals. What we call "pure vegetarians" are only second-hand *meat*ers.

I am indebted to the distinguished champion tennis-player, diet-reformer, and restaurator Eustace Miles, for the name "Meaters" to designate those who eat meat; and I have coined the term "Mealers" to stand for those who take only first-hand earth-fruit products for their nutrition, disregarding the fact that all are *meal*ers who take *meals* of victuals. To offset this addition to the vocabulary, it would do no harm to drop off the use of "Meals" and "Victuals," leaving "Meal" to mean only one thing; viz., ground cereals or vegetables.[P]

One of the details of carefulness in Fletcherism is expressed in the statement that we should not *pro*scribe as food anything that Nature permits to be utilized as food; but the same carefulness prescribes that we do not *pre*scribe it as food for everybody all of the time. Everything in its proper time and place is one of the common-sense rules of the system.

Captain Amundsen and his comrades, as I have already observed, were quite justified in devouring their faithful and friendly sledge dogs when necessary to preserve their own lives. I have the acquaintance of a collie dog whom I love devotedly; and I say "whom" appropriately because he is as intelligent as I am, and far more consistent in his habits of orderliness and naturalness. He is a real gentleman at all times and as good a Fletcherite when the food substance and occasion demand as I am. He has learned to eat and enjoy apples and no one could give more careful mouth-treatment to some sorts of food than Bruce. I am sure that he would want me to eat him if I needed him to preserve my life, just as unselfishly as the Japanese soldiers, and more recently the Balkanese soldiers, gave their lives for their causes. Whether I would eat him or not I cannot say, and I do not know if he would have similar consideration or otherwise for me.

I merely use this illustration as an aside in consideration of the question of flesh eating on emergency or sentimental grounds. Nature permits Bruce and me to eat each other, and if we managed it skilfully we could attack each other's extremities at the same time, as long as we did not encroach on our vital machinery, and really eat each other up, as young lovers would like to do.

Thus much for sentiment. We are subsisting on ourselves all of the time; we can nourish ourselves at the expense of each other if we will.

We can eat human flesh as nourishingly as we can a Spring chicken, and if we do not know what we are eating, Nature will say us never "No," but there are other considerations more practical for every-day consideration. These are: physiological and economic expediency.

MEAT AND URIC ACID

In the thorough investigation that Dr. Hindhede, of Copenhagen, has conducted for the past few years, and in which I have assisted, I have followed the quest with eagerness because of the thoroughness of it. It has been proven that very little protein or nitrogen is needed for the human body even under strain of hardest physical or mental activity. On the other hand, it has been found that any appreciable excess of protein or nitrogen results in both uric acid secretion and increased blood-pressure, meaning, in all probability, finally fatal strain on the organism. It has also been demonstrated that it is almost impossible to take the leaner meats without getting more protein or nitrogen than the body needs.

It is quite easy to get excessive protein and nitrogen from vegetable, farinaceous, and hen-fruit material, and cheeses are richer than anything in these "strong" food ingredients; but these are not such subtle foolers of the appetite as meats done up in spicy gravies and accompanied by appetising fats.

I purposely avoid giving any figures relative to the food values under mention because the first rule of Fletcherism in connection with the selection and intake of food is to leave that entirely to appetite, working intelligently and normally in relation to the food that is available at the moment.

To my thinking, the most important consideration is economy, not alone of the money cost of food, but economy of energy-consumption within the body. There may be times when economy of money-cost means much to persons struggling to lay aside an independent competency for the purchase of leisure in old age, or for insurance against becoming a burden upon others; and this is sure to happen to all who are not cursed by the handicap of money inheritance. But it is the internal economy of the body that counts for most in estimating values. There is no doubt but what flesh food is a stimulant of the same or similar character of alcohol. Both of these subtle agents of intemperance invite the starting and accumulation of vicious cycles or circles (swirls) of over-stimulation that have one bad effect, at least, on the comfort and efficiency of the muscular tissues. They facilitate fatigue and "that tired feeling," and also may result in contingent "soreness" of muscle after unusual exercise.

Faithful Fletcherizing has resulted in regulating these matters in a way that is nothing less than marvellous until the reasons are revealed.

Not only does observance of the habit and practice which Mr. Rockefeller has condensed into thirty-three words, including several repetitions for emphasis, result in settling the questions of appropriateness, economy, emergencies, and comfort in general between the *Meat*ers and the *Meal*ers; between the mixed *Meat*ers and *Meal*ers; and between the Physiology and Psychology of normality;

and which Mr. Rockefeller calls "Fletcherizing," but a whole lot of beneficent cycles or circles (rhythms) of profitable felicities are set in motion.

TO SUM UP

The *Meal*ers have the advantage of the argument in that they are always on the safer side of prudence, and there is no real deprivation involved in the experiment.

At the present moment I am, personally, still in the experimental field as regards everything that Nature permits as food or drink. There is one point that vegetarianism has not satisfactorily answered as yet. The great majority of conscientious vegetarians have not the pink complexion that is usually reckoned as a sign of beauty or robustness, but I have known one, Frederick Madsen (Madsen the Faithful), an assistant of Dr. Hindhede in Copenhagen, to subsist on potatoes and butter, or margarine, alone, for three hundred days consecutively, stopping only because the potatoes to be had in the market were not as good as desired, and he lost none of his pinky-pinkness of complexion of the richest Scandinavian brilliancy. I have done the same for four months with similar results of retention of pinkness of complexion. Another question is: Does pinkness indicate health? It is not the necessity of health among Latins and bronzed Orientals, but it underlies the bronze exterior in even African Negroes, if they are healthy. Sallow is the reverse of healthy in proportion to the sallowness, as a usual thing.

Just here is where the efficacy of careful eating, which has been formulated as Fletcherism, comes into service most agreeably to make life really worth living and actually one continuous festival of usefulness and pleasure. It is only once formed into a habit and set to working automatically under the direction of Appetite, Taste, Feeling, Instinct, and the other attributes of sub-conscious Intelligence.

It will be noted that Mr. Rockefeller, in his recent pithy, gisty utterance relative to the merits of Fletcherizing, makes no mention of the kind of food to be recommended. Happily, as far as I know, he is not in the food business, has no connection with any special food supply, and cannot recommend any of the products of petroleum as food or drink. He should be absolutely unprejudiced in his judgment, and seven or eight years of recuperative experience, similar to mine of a longer period, is material for judgment and recommendation.

Some years ago there was born in me the ambition to formulate the rules of economic procedure in securing optimum nutrition in a space of not more than ten pages of coarse print that mothers, teachers, and children of primary school age could understand as easy as the noses on their faces. Mr. Rockefeller has "beat me out" in brevity by several lengths. He has made the revelation with the lucky number of thirty-three words, and left room for a final remark full of scriptural tone, as is his wont.

PROFITABLE ECONOMY

There is one argument in favour of a meatless diet that appeals to everybody, and that is the economy and cleanliness of it. In Professor Irving Fisher's classic investigation to test the merits of Fletcherism it was proven that careful attention to the mastication, insalivation, and enjoyment of food while in the mouth, and swallowing only in response to a strong invitation to swallow, and removing from the mouth whatever remainder that did not practically *swallow itself,* a net gain of approximately 40 per cent. was achieved without any attempt at economy. The saving was in the money cost alone, and it came from more and more inclination towards farinaceous and vegetable foods and away from more expensive meat.

This form of saving is very telling. Dr. Francis E. Clark, founder and permanent president of the great International Christian Endeavour organization, noticed a reduction of one-third in the food expenses of his family. The health officer of a suburb of Hamburg accomplished a saving of two thousand marks a year in his family of three without other assistance than careful eating and an inclination towards non-flesh food material. The "Poor White Trash" community in America, before mentioned, saved an average of three dollars a month each, three thousand dollars a month among a thousand members of the community, and the missionary workers who taught them to Fletcherize save half of the cost of their sustenance. Accompanying all of this wonderful economy was an immunity from the ordinary illnesses that was worth more than the money saving.

In the Rockefeller family any decrease in the cost of food is a negligible quantity in comparison with the total expenses, but seven years of immunity from indigestion and replacing the demon with good golf-health form have been worth more than millions of money.

APPENDIX

WAS LUIGI CORNARO RIGHT?

>A PAPER READ BEFORE THE PHYSIOLOGICAL SECTION OF THE BRITISH MEDICAL ASSOCIATION, AUGUST, 1901, BY ERNEST VAN SOMEREN

Mr. President and Gentlemen:

Being a general practitioner, it is with some trepidation and an apology that I present myself before this section. The reasons for my doing so are: First, that I believe that a hitherto unsuspected reflex in deglutition has come to light which has an important bearing on health, the prevention of disease and on metabolism. Second, that any theory whatever, based on a possible physiological function, claiming to diminish, as this does, the amount of sickness and suffering now existent, should have serious investigation. Third, that I desire to enlist your skilled help in the consideration of the theories I have doubtless crudely erected on my premise.

According to the "Encyclopædia Britannica," "Luigi Cornaro (1467-1566) was a Venetian nobleman, famous for his treatises on a temperate life. From some dishonesty on the part of his relatives, he was deprived of his rank and induced to retire to Padua, where he acquired the experience in regard to food and regimen which he has detailed in his work. In his youth he lived freely, but after a severe illness at the age of forty, he began under medical advice gradually to reduce his diet. For some time he restricted himself to a daily allowance of 12 ozs. of solid food and 14 ozs. of wine. Later in life he still farther reduced his bill of fare, and he found that he could support his life and strength with no more solid meat than an egg a day. So much habituated did he become to this simple diet that when he was about seventy years of age the addition, by way of experiment, of 2 ozs. a day had nearly proved fatal. At the age of eighty-three he wrote his treatise on the 'Sure and Certain Method of Attaining a Long and Healthful Life.' And this work was followed by three others on the same subject, composed at the ages of eighty-six, ninety-one, and ninety-five, respectively. 'They are written,' says Addison ('Spectator,' No. 195), 'with such a spirit of cheerfulness, religion, and good sense, as are the natural concomitants of temperance, and sobriety.' He died at the age of ninety-eight." Some say of 103!

Now, was Luigi Cornaro right? Did he make use of a physiological process unknown to us of the value of which he was not cognisant? To live to an advanced age, must we be as temperate as he, reducing the quantity of our food to a minimum required by Nature?

That we all eat more than we can assimilate is unquestionable. How can we determine the right quantity? Instinct *should* guide us, but an abnormal appetite often leads us astray. Nature's plans are perfect if her laws are obeyed. Disease follows disobedience. Wherein do we disobey?

We live *not* upon what we eat, but upon what we digest; then why should undigested food, recognisable as such, be deemed a normal constituent of our solid egesta?

Something like the following must be a common experience to general practitioners, especially to those practising on the Continent. The patient comes to see us and volunteers the information that he or she has the "gout," "rheumatic gout," or "dyspepsia." Symptoms are asked for. The case is gone into carefully for causation. An appropriate diet and an appropriate bottle of medicine prescribed. As the patient leaves the room, we may, or may not, call attention to the fact that both teeth and saliva are meant to be used. The patient returns, better, *in statu quo*, or worse. If better, he remains so while under treatment, and relapses when he returns to ordinary habits. If unaffected, or worse, we try again and again, until we despair, then take or send him to a consultant. Temporary benefit, possibly owing to renewed hope, results; but finally the unfortunate gets used to his sufferings, and, if he can afford it, is sent to join the innumerable hosts that wander from one Bad to another, all Europe over, trying, praising, and damning each in turn. Their manner of living is, of course, at fault. Nature never intended that man should be perpetually on a special diet and hugging a bottle of medicine, nor did she ordain that he should go wandering over the map of Europe drinking purgative and other waters.

Though early yet to speak with certain voice, it would seem that we are provided with a Guard, reliance on which protects us from the results of mal-nutrition. There seems to be placed in the fauces and the back of the mouth a Monitor to warn us what we ought to swallow and when we ought to swallow it. The good offices of this Monitor we have suppressed by habits of too rapid eating, acquired in infancy or youth.

Last November my attention was called by Mr. Horace Fletcher, an American author living in Venice, to the discovery in himself of a curious inability to swallow, and a closing of the throat against food, unless it had been completely masticated. My informant stated that he noticed this peculiarity after he had begun to excessively insalivate his food, both liquid and solid, until all its original taste had been removed from it. Any tasteless residue in the mouth, being refused by the fauces, required a *forced* muscular effort to swallow. He further told me that since adopting this method of eating he had been cured of two maladies, adjudged chronic, the suffering from which rendered him ineligible for Life Insurance. His weight now became reduced from 205 lbs. to 165 lbs. He had practised no abstemiousness, had indulged his appetite, both as to selection and to quantity, without restraint, and for the last three years had enjoyed perfect health.

After his cure, he was accepted without difficulty for insurance, the last examination finding him an unusually healthy subject for his age. Having leisure, he had spent three years in investigating the cause of his cure, had pursued experiments upon others, and had extended his inquiries, both in America and Europe, until our meeting in Venice. He had also published a statement and inquiry in book form, entitled "Glutton or Epicure," which had been reviewed by the "Lancet."

For nearly a year I also had been experimenting on myself and others with various diets, and was ready to believe that in the manner of taking food and not altogether in its varying *matter* lay perhaps its protean effects on our system. I at once adopted the same method of eating. At the end of six weeks, I noticed that not only did the fauces refuse to allow of the passage of imperfectly prepared food, but that such food was returned from the back to the front of the mouth by an involuntary, though eventually controllable, muscular effort taking place in the reverse direction to that occurring at the inception of deglutition.

What actually happens is this: Food, as it is masticated, slowly passes to the back of the mouth, and collects in the glosso-epiglottidean folds, where it remains in contact with the mucous membrane containing the sensory end-organs of taste. If it be properly reduced by the saliva it is allowed to pass the fauces,—a truly involuntary act of deglutition occurring. Let the food, however, be too rapidly passed back to these folds, *i. e.*, before complete reduction takes place, and the reflex muscular movement above referred to occurs. The process of this reflex is as follows: The tip of the tongue is involuntarily fixed at the backs and bases of the lower central incisor teeth by the anterior fibres of the geniohyoglossi muscles. With this fixed point as fulcrum, the lower and middle fibres of these muscles, aided by those of the stylohyoid and styloglossi muscles raise the hyoid bone, straighten out the glosso-epiglottidean folds, passing their contents forward, by the fauces, the opening of which is closed by approximation of its pillars and contraction of the superior constrictor. The tongue, arched postero-anteriorly by the geniohyoglossi, palato, and styloglossi muscles, laterally, by its own intrinsic muscles, is approximated to the fauces, soft and hard palates in turn, and thus, the late contents of the glosso-epiglottidean folds are returned to the front of the mouth for further reduction by the saliva preparatory to deglutition.

The word reduction is used for the reason that all foods tested, without exception, give an acid reaction to litmus, when served at table. The reflex muscular movement occurs in the writer's case from five to ten times during the mastication of each mouthful of food, according to its quantity and its degree of sapidity. As often as it recurs, the returned food continues to give an acid reaction, while food allowed to pass the fauces is alkaline.

Saliva, flowing in response to the stimulation of taste, seems more alkaline than that secreted in answer to mechanical tasteless stimulation. It is found that the removal of original taste from any given bolus of food coincides with cessation of salivary flow and complete alkaline reduction. The fibre of meat, gristle, connective tissue, the husk of coarse bread and cellulose of vegetables are carefully separated by the tongue and buccal muscles and rejected by the fauces. To swallow any of these necessitates a *forced* muscular effort, which is abnormal.

Adult man was not originally intended to take his nourishment in a liquid form, consequently all liquids having taste, such as soup, milk, tea, coffee, cocoa, and the various forms of alcohol, must be treated as sapid solids and insalivated by holding them in the mouth, moving the tongue gently, with straight up and down masticatory movements, until their taste be removed. Water, not having taste, needs no insalivation and is readily accepted by the fauces.

In explanation of the phenomenon described, the following theory is advanced: The fauces back of the tongue, epiglottis, in short, those mucous surfaces in which are placed the sensory end-organs of taste and "taste buds" (the distribution of which, by the way, has yet to be explained), that these surfaces, readily becoming accustomed to an alkaline contact by excessive insalivation and consequent complete alkaline reduction of the food, afterwards resent an acid contact and express their resentment by throwing off the cause of offence by the muscles underlying them.

This phenomenon must not be confused with the cases of rumination and regurgitation, which from time to time are recorded. The food in this case is not swallowed, nor does it pass any point from which it can be regurgitated. Eighty-one individuals of different nationalities and from several classes of society whom we have studied are now in conscious possession of their reflexes. These seem readily educated back to normal functions by all who seriously and patiently adopt the habit of what seems only at first to be excessive insalivation.

The dictum "bite your food well" that we so often use, has no meaning to those suffering from the results of mal-assimilation and mal-nutrition, especially should they have few or no teeth of their own. I make so bold as to state that dyspepsia *et morbi hujus generis omnis* will cease to exist if patients be persuaded to bite their food until its original taste disappears, and it is carried away by involuntary deglutition.

The important point of the whole question seems to be this alkaline reduction of of acid food before it passes on to meet subsequent digestive processes elsewhere, which then become alternately acid and alkaline.

In the first few months of infant life, when saliva is not secreted, Nature ordains that mammary secretion be alkaline. With the eruption of teeth come an abundant flow of saliva and a synchronous infantile capacity for managing other foods. This flow of saliva depends on a thorough demand and use to maintain its generous supply. It is just at this time that children learn to bolt their food,—the demand fails, with a consequent detriment to the salivary glands, digestive processes, and the system generally.

A, B, C, and D were placed on an absolute milk diet. A drank his milk in the ordinary way, and at the end of three days begged to discontinue the experiment owing to disgust at the monotony of the diet. B, C, and D continued the experiment for seventeen days, insalivating the milk, but to a varying extent, B the least and D the most. Though D took most milk, he excreted least solid egesta, C excreting less than B. Can one infer that increased insalivation of a non-starchy food insured its better digestion and assimilation? Each subject took as much milk only as his appetite demanded, D taking the most, which never exceeded two litres daily. The weights of the subjects after the usual sudden drop of the first three days remained remarkably even until the end of the experiment. B, C, and D all relished the diet, and it satisfied the requirements of their appetites, but they experienced an increasing monotony.

As long ago as the seventeenth century, before the transformation of matter into energy by the animal organism, known as Metabolism, was understood, the fact was recognised that by the lungs, kidneys, skin, and intestines, substances no longer useful to the organism were eliminated, the retention of which proved harmful. The nature of these substances was unknown, but it was noted that however much the food was increased the weight of the body remained the same. In other words, a state of complete nutritive equilibrium was maintained.

The following table contains the *résumé* of two experiments in which a state of complete nutritive equilibrium was maintained by individuals of about the same weight, on widely different quantities of food similar in quality. The subjects of the experiments were a laboratory assistant of Dr. Snyder, of the U. S. Department of Agriculture, and the writer. The experiment of the former was made primarily to show the relative digestibility of the several articles of diet, potatoes, eggs, milk, and cream:

	Dr. Snyder's Experiment. Published in Bulletin 43	Writer's Experiment.
Age of subject	22 years	30 years
Duration of experiment	4 1/3 days	5 days
Number of meals	13	10
Weight at beginning	62.5 kilos	57.3 kilos
Weight at end	62.6 kilos	57.5 kilos
Potatoes (daily average)	1587.6 grammes	159.4 grammes
Eggs (daily average)	411.08 grammes	124.7 grammes
Milk (daily average)	710 c.c.	710 c.c.
Cream (daily average)	237 c.c.	237 c.c.
Daily urine	1108 grammes	1098 grammes
Daily fæces	204 grammes	18.9 grammes

The daily diet of Dr. Snyder's subject consisted of three and one-half pounds of potatoes, eight eggs, a pint and a half of milk, and half a pint of cream. The writer's diet of twelve ounces of solid food (like Luigi Cornaro) consisted of three eggs, the remainder of the twelve ounces in potatoes, and an equal quantity of similar liquid food to that taken by Dr. Snyder's subject. The exercise of the laboratory assistant comprised his daily routine of laboratory work, while that of the writer consisted of six sets of tennis, or an hour and a half on horseback, with an hour to an hour and a half's walk or climb daily, in addition to much reading and writing.

In each case complete nutritive equilibrium was maintained, although the author subsisted on three-seventeenths of the solid food taken by the other subject.

Again, cannot one infer that better assimilation and less waste resulted from the better preparation of the smaller quantity of food by insalivation? Surely, too, there must be less daily strain on the intestinal canal, and body generally, in getting rid of 18.9 grammes of inoffensive dry waste, than in getting rid of 204 grammes of humid, decomposing, and offensive matter.

"Considerable importance has been attached to the normal action of the bacteria in the intestines; and it has even been supposed that the presence of bacteria is essential to life. Such a view has recently been shown to be erroneous by an elaborate and painstaking research carried out by Nuttall and Thierfelder, who obtained ripe fœtal guinea-pigs by means of Cæsarean section carried out under strict antiseptic precautions. They introduced the animals immediately into an asceptic chamber through which a current of filtered air was aspirated, and fed them hourly on sterilised milk day and night for over eight days.

"The animals lived, and throve, and increased as much in weight as healthy normal animals subjected to a similar diet for the purpose of controlling the results. Microscopic examination at the end of the experiment showed that the alimentary canal contained no bacteria of any kind, nor could cultures of any kind be obtained from it.

"The same authors, in a subsequent paper, described the extension of their research to vegetable food. This was also digested in the absence of bacteria. Under such conditions cellulose was not attacked. Hence they consider that the chief function of this material is to give bulk and proper consistency to the food so as to suit the conditions of herbivorous digestion." (Schäfer's "Text-Book of Physiology," vol. i., p. 465.)

Now, inasmuch as bacterial digestion has no place in the animal economy, surely it can only occur at the expense of the organism?

Can micro-organic action take place in the intestines without the production of toxins and the consequent absorption of these toxins into the blood?

We know that the metabolism of a cell is determined by the general physical environment of the whole organism, by supplies of oxygen and water, on nervous impulses, and, what chiefly concerns this argument, on the nature and amount of the pabulum supplied to it. This pabulum is derived from the alimentary canal.

Are not even those of us who may be enjoying seemingly the best of health supplying to our tissues pabulum containing mild toxins, thus causing an increased katabolic action to occur in each individual cell of our bodies?

Are not the blood elements, floating in a plasma containing such toxins, rendered resistant, weaker, less capable of fulfilling their functions as carriers and combatants of disease?

Are not their and our lives, in consequence, more painful and shorter than they need be?

Would not the elimination of these toxins render us less liable to disease? And is not their presence an important element in predisposition to disease?

When this reflex is restored micro-organisms get no further than the stomach. They are destroyed there by the acid gastric juices, then only stimulated to their full and normal secretion by the presence of a sufficiency of alkaline substance. Undigested matter having been eliminated, micro-organisms, still existing in the intestines, deprived of their means of subsistence, decrease, and, in time, may cease to exist. The body no longer absorbs the toxins these produced. To this fact may be ascribed the increase of mental energy, the general physical betterment, the cessation of morbid cravings for food and drink and of those of a sexual nature, which are noticed and experienced.

What has just been stated is based not entirely on experimental evidence but somewhat upon inference. The inference seems justified because the excreta, more especially of the intestines, but also of the kidneys and skin, become almost odourless and entirely inoffensive. The solid egesta are voided thickly covered with mucus, leaving the end of the bowel dry and clean. The sense of cleanliness can only then be appreciated to the full, for it is internal as well as external. *Flatus* is no longer produced. The urine is inoffensive and seems to be materially changed in quality, as shown by chemical analysis. Uric acid, the chlorides, and, more markedly, aromatic sulphates are reduced in quantity.

Owing to deliberation in eating, necessitated by this new habit, satiety occurs on the ingestion of considerably less food. By carefully studying one's self I believe it possible to cultivate an instinct which will regulate not only the quantity but the quality of food that the body may need, and that in the *normal health* of a full-grown body, no more food either in quantity or quality should be supplied than suffices to supply diurnal waste. Any excess must result in pathological processes.

Although there results enhanced pleasure in the taking of all foods, rich and simple, and especially in the appreciation of good wines, the quantities of these foods and beverages that suffice to fully satisfy the appetite are much smaller than before, while there is a marked preference for the simpler kinds of food. The writer now can imagine no more pleasurable meal than one consisting of good brown bread, eggs, butter, cheese, and cream. These, with fresh vegetables and a very little fruit, form his staple diet. This tendency and preference for simple foods is the general experience among those who have recovered their reflexes of deglutition.

Following on the ingestion of a lessened quantity of food and on its better assimilation, there is less waste, the egesta are voided less frequently, sometimes only once in five to eight days.

The lower bowel is not the reservoir it formerly was. So hæmorrhoids cease from troubling and constipation cannot exist. For this same reason the body, at the beginning of the practice, commences to approximate to its normal weight, increasing or decreasing as the individual's environment demands.

A few more words only need be said. It has been easy to state the results of experiments and observations: but the acquiring of this new reflex, while pursuing daily occupations, is not easy, and needs more than a little patience and much serious thought. The habits of a lifetime cannot be changed in a few days or weeks. The shortest time in which the reflex has been re-established is four weeks, and this only by avoiding conversation at meal-time and concentrating the attention on keeping the food in the mouth until complete alkaline reduction has taken place and sapidity has disappeared.

In closing I wish to maintain as a fact, gentlemen, of the truth of which you will only be convinced by actual experience, that by the restoration of this reflex and in complete dependence on its use, there lies true health, the establishment of a condition of stable nutrition and the possible abrogation of two great predisposing factors of disease, mal-assimilation and mal-nutrition. Unless there be among you, as in the "Cities of the Plain," a parlous minority who possess this reflex and take your food as you ought, none of you are in the enjoyment of such health as you might have. A like punishment will be meted out to you as was visited on those cities, for you will all be consumed long before your day by the unnecessary combustion in your bodies caused by the circulation in them of toxins, the product of undigested and decomposing food.

The writer, bearing in mind the warning suggested by the Frenchman whose donkey died as soon as he had reduced his food to a single wisp of straw, finds that he is taking less and less food. While his mind is open as to his arriving at the final diet of Luigi Cornaro, yet it is easily conceivable that living a similar life of retirement in a placid environment, it would be quite possible to do as he did. Hence the title of this paper and the queries at the commencement.

The objects in publishing and distributing this paper are twofold: to make the subject as widely known as possible, and to solicit the aid of colleagues in investigating it more fully.

There is ready at the service of the general practitioner an important and potential therapeutic agent in the saliva of his patients and in the use *ad finem* of their salivary digestions.

Editor's notes. (1) Confirmatory evidence of the correctness of the deductions made in this paper has begun to come in from many professional sources and notably from a famous child specialist who avers that children would follow the natural requirements in eating were it not for artificial food, bad example, and bad teaching.

(2) In a report of a paper read before the *Société de Biologie*, Paris, France, March 15th, 1902, by M. Max Marckwald, of Kreuznach, "ON DIGESTION OF MILK IN THE STOMACH OF FULL-GROWN DOGS," the following appears: "Hence these experiments confirm those of Horace Fletcher and Ernest H. Van Someren on the importance of prolonged mastication" (*translation*). Referring, as the latter statement does, to mastication (insalivation) of liquid, it gives an important suggestion relative to some probable causes of uncertain or defective digestion in human nutrition.

www.ingramcontent.com/pod-product-compliance
Lightning Source LLC
Chambersburg PA
CBHW070914180526
45168CB00005B/2009